The politics of health promotion

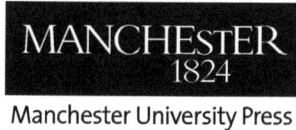

Manchester University Press

The politics of health promotion

Case studies from Denmark and England

Peter Triantafillou and Naja Vucina

Manchester University Press

Copyright © Peter Triantafillou and Naja Vucina 2018

The right of Peter Triantafillou and Naja Vucina to be identified as the authors of this work has been asserted by them in accordance with the Copyright, Designs and Patents Act 1988.

Published by Manchester University Press
Altrincham Street, Manchester M1 7JA
www.manchesteruniversitypress.co.uk

British Library Cataloguing-in-Publication Data
A catalogue record for this book is available from the British Library

ISBN 978 1 5261 0052 8 hardback

First published 2018

The publisher has no responsibility for the persistence or accuracy of URLs for any external or third-party internet websites referred to in this book, and does not guarantee that any content on such websites is, or will remain, accurate or appropriate.

Typeset by Out of House Publishing
Printed by Lightning Source

Contents

Acknowledgements vi

Introduction 1
1 Critical studies of the politics of public health promotion 13
2 Governing public health in England and Denmark 33
3 Fighting obesity in England 59
4 Governing obesity in Denmark 79
5 Promoting recovery in England 99
6 Promoting recovery in Denmark 115
Conclusion 133

Bibliography 146
Index 168

Acknowledgements

We would like to acknowledge the highly useful comments and suggestions provided by the anonymous referees. We also want to acknowledge the support of Tony Mason and Robert Byron for managing the editorial process in a highly professional fashion, as well as the efforts of the whole team at Manchester University Press.

Introduction

The NHS needs a far more proactive and preventative approach to reduce the long term impact for people experiencing mental health problems and for their families, and to reduce costs for the NHS and emergency services. (Mental Health Taskforce, 2016, p. 4)

To be successful, a comprehensive long-term strategy to tackle obesity must act in two complementary ways to achieve and maintain a healthy population weight distribution. First, an environment that supports and facilitates healthy choices must be actively established and maintained. Second, individuals need to be encouraged to desire, seek and make different choices, recognizing that they make decisions as part of families or groups and that individual behaviour is 'cued' by the behaviours of others, including organisational behaviours and other wider influences. (Butland et al., 2007, p. 122)

The inhabitants of most OECD countries tend to regard state intervention in the everyday lives of individual citizens and in society at large with a certain scepticism. At the very least governments and public authorities in so-called liberal democracies are expected to come up with quite convincing moral arguments to justify interventions that go beyond protecting basic civil and political rights. One does not have to be a libertarian to acknowledge that state power may have quite far-reaching implications for our everyday life and that the orchestration and mobilization of such powers calls for critical attention. Notwithstanding liberal concerns over state power (and the many inbuilt mechanisms in liberal democracies to account for and regulate its use), there is an area in which most liberal democracies seem to be very tolerant in the use of direct state power: the governing of public health and the vigour and quality of the lives of individuals and populations seem to constitute a case in which liberal concerns over state interventions at times seem less adamant.

For more than a century, industrially developed states have contributed to the establishment of comprehensive and widely available health

2 The politics of health promotion

services, such as hospitals, clinics, general practitioners, home nurses, and community health centres (Starr, 1982; Blank and Burau, 2014). We have also seen the development of large-scale physical infrastructure interventions to ensure sewage treatment, clean water, and waste management (Corbin, 1986). While our growing cities may seem chaotic, the design of housing, streets, and squares has been strictly regulated since the end of the nineteenth century to ensure hygiene, clean water, and reasonably clean air with a view towards ensuring public health (Latour, 1988). The state then has intervened extensively in society in the name of public health since the nineteenth century.

Michel Foucault used the term biopower to designate the modern state's responsibility for ensuring the vigour and quality of the population inhabiting its (the state's) territory (Foucault, 1978, pp. 139–141). Sovereign, state power would now be used not so much to take life but to invest in life and its quality. Moreover, during the nineteenth and twentieth centuries a series of regulatory interventions, relying less on sovereign power of commands and interdictions but more on indirect forms of power, were launched to promote personal conduct and physical spaces more conducive to public health. Yet these regulatory interventions targeting both individuals and the population have generally been limited by liberal concerns over excessive state interventions (Osborne, 1997). The aspirations of the programmes seeking to cure and prevent illness have usually been tamed by institutionalized norms of civil and political rights protecting individuals and society at large from instances of state power and other powers not grounded in constitutional or legal regulations. Thus, both curative and preventive strategies have usually targeted the health of individuals and populations in a voluntary and/or indirect way. The curative services offered by hospitals, general practitioners, and others are just that: offers. Unless you have a highly contagious and dangerous disease, no one will force you to see a doctor. The preventive strategies seeking to promote hygiene by constructing sewage systems, securing clean drinking water, organizing waste management systems, and regulating housing design and construction all work indirectly. They modify the physical environment of citizens to make this more hygienic and healthy. These changes to the physical environment may alter the everyday conduct of citizens quite significantly, but this happens indirectly.

Of course, Western societies – corresponding roughly to the existing OECD countries – have seen the use of direct and even coercive forms of preventive interventions in the name of the population's vigour and quality. All over these societies, the emergence of the eugenic movement in the interwar period resulted in various public interventions seeking to protect the quality of the stock by trying to reduce the reproduction of the physically and mentally unfit, culminating with the Nazi extermination programme to ensure the purity of the Aryan race. The eugenic movement – at least in its negative form – has so far served as a political warning of just how wrong things can go when sovereign state power is mobilized in the name of the population's vigour and quality. Thus, Western societies have been reluctant to use coercive means and to use interventions directly targeting and modifying behaviour or conduct. This may be about to change.

While coercion is hardly on the contemporary public health agendas of these countries, they have witnessed the emergence of an approach that urges state power to be both intensified in order to reach ever deeper into the personal dispositions of individuals and to be extended to reach into ever more parts of the social environment shaping the choice and conduct of citizens. Thus, under the broad heading of health promotion, we have seen the unfolding of a wide range of new ideas, strategies, programmes, and techniques that are trying not to cure illness but to promote health (World Health Organization, 1986, 1998). The WHO's Health for All strategy adopted in the mid-1980s seems to have contributed significantly to the framing of health promotion ideas and strategies in many OECD countries. To get the gist of the new approach, it may be worth quoting the WHO's Ottawa Charter at some length:

> [H]ealth promotion demands coordinated action by all concerned: by governments, by health and other social and economic sectors, by nongovernmental and voluntary organizations, by industry and by the media ... Health promotion goes beyond health care. It puts health on the agenda of policy makers in all sectors and at all levels, directing them to be aware of the health consequences of their decisions and to accept their responsibilities for health ... Health promotion policy requires the identification of obstacles to the adoption of healthy public policies in non-health sectors and ways of removing them. The aim must be to make the healthy choice the easier choice for policymakers as well. (World Health Organization, 1986, p. 2)

In the following years, most countries in Europe, North America, and the Antipodes, and several countries in Asia, have designed strategies and launched programmes that seek to promote health and to prevent, rather than cure, illness (Blank and Burau, 2014, pp. 208–213). The distinction between health promotion and curing of illness may seem an insignificant one, but the political implications of the two conceptions and the strategies they imply are substantial. The cure of illness is a relatively narrow and well-defined political enterprise; health promotion is not. To cure illness is limited to specific target groups (those deemed ill); health promotion targets each and every citizen. A cure has a start and an end; health promotion is a never-ending process in as much as it is always possible for everyone – even the most apparently healthy person – to further improve her healthiness or vigour. Health promotion then is really not about curing diseases or even about preventing diseases. While the promotion of health should, according to its own success criteria, be able to reduce the likelihood that a person falls ill and thereby be preventive, its ambition goes further than the prevention of illness. As hammered out over and again by the WHO, national health authorities, and a number of health professionals, the ambition of health promotion is not only to reduce the risk of falling ill but also to augment the health and vigour of a person and of the population at large. This implies that each and every one starts reflecting on their own health, their habits of dieting and physical exercise, and further, as we shall see in the following chapters, that our social environments and relations are shaped in ways that are conducive to the choice of a healthy lifestyle. In this sense, health promotion goes much farther than any hitherto existing preventive strategy, including the infamous eugenic movement.

In the somatic area, obesity has become a phenomenon of acute political concern. Until recently, obesity was not regarded as an illness. The populations of many OECD countries are living an increasingly sedentary life and consuming increasing amounts of high-fat and high-sugar food products. Accordingly, the prevalence of overweight and obese people has increased more or less steadily. Today, medical experts are debating whether obesity should be considered a disease. However, they agree that obesity significantly enhances the risk of contracting so-called lifestyle diseases, such as diabetes, a wide range of cardiovascular diseases, orthopaedic diseases, and certain forms of cancer (World Health Organization, 2016). This has caused some US medical experts to regard obesity as a threat to national economic sustainability (Olshansky, Passaro, Hershow, Layden, and Carnes, 2005). They expect that obesity among American children and youth will dramatically increase health costs and erode the tax base, as the capacity of the obese to remain in employment will drop.

Partly informed by this medical knowledge, we have seen the emergence of a wide array of health promotion interventions that work neither by curing diseases nor even by modifying the physical environment – though we find both these types of interventions too. These new interventions are targeting the individual and the social environment in order to make people adopt a healthier lifestyle. The individualizing interventions include fitness courses, therapeutic procedures, cookery programmes, obesity camps, self-esteem techniques, and workplace gymnastics (Ayo, 2012). In a few instances, such as in Singapore, these interventions include mandatory physical training programmes for obese children (Foo, Vijaya, Sloan, and Ling, 2013). We have also seen the emergence of interventions targeting the social environment of the obese and the general population. This includes the forging of networks or joined-up government between schools, workplaces, sports clubs, community centres, and various voluntary organizations on the one hand,

and hospitals, clinicians, general practitioners, and municipal health services on the other (Blank and Burau, 2014, pp. 217–221). Network or joined-up governance is invoked here to make it easier for individuals, families, and groups to choose and actually live a healthier life (Vucina, 2014, pp. 164–189). The WHO has encouraged such comprehensive strategies based on extensive cooperation between public agencies, and between such agencies and all parts of civil society in order to reach not only the obese, but also those who at a later stage in their life may gain excessive weight, in particular children and young people (WHO Regional Office for Europe, 2006).

The development of health promotion interventions emphasizing lifestyle changes may be seen as the obvious or natural response to the growing prevalence of obesity and the diseases it may induce. However, on closer inspection this response is not so obvious. Firstly, there is strong medical evidence suggesting that the risks from being overweight or slightly obese are negligible and in some cases it may even be beneficial (Flegal, Kit, Orpana, and Graubard, 2013). Secondly, health promotion interventions are extremely costly. In fact, it has been estimated that the costs of obesity control outweigh the benefits (van Baal et al., 2008). Thirdly, and most importantly from the point of view of this book, health promotion interventions interfere very directly in the everyday life of people, something that usually arouses suspicion and resistance. While we often accept the right of public authorities to step in and regulate everyday behaviour in cases of contagious diseases, in the case of most other diseases liberal rationalities tend to prevail, in the sense that people are given a choice of whether they want to receive treatment or not. In the case of obesity, which many medical experts do not even regard as a disease, there seems to be an increasing consensus on the need for extensive interventions. This acceptance of public intervention to control obesity seems even more curious if we consider that most interventions target not only the obese but all those at risk at becoming overweight or obese (i.e. everyone).

Within mental health we have seen the emergence of so-called community psychiatry or community mental health and outpatient treatment. This reflects the de-institutionalization of the treatment of people suffering from a wide range of mental illnesses. During the 1970s and 1980s, many patients were moved from the ambit of the asylums and mental hospitals to more or less well-integrated networks of psychiatric programmes, general practitioners, municipal services, and specialized housing projects that seek to create a life close to 'normal' (Castel, Castel, and Lovell, 1982, pp. 162–169; Grob, 1991). Apart from saving money on running costly mental hospitals, the proponents of community health services argue that many patients are cured more effectively outside of hospitals and that even those who are never fully cured may experience a richer and fuller life outside the confines of the mental institutions (World Health Organization, 2001, 2007). Thus, the basic rationale of community mental health interventions is really to empower the mentally ill via the enabling institutions and services offered by the community.

The biomedical approach to a number of mental diseases, including schizophrenia, changed quite significantly during this period of de-institutionalization. In particular, the emergence of recovery as a strategy emphasizing the enhanced ability of the patient to cope with her symptoms, rather than eradicating these, stands out. Recovery is the label for a wide range of relatively recent schemes, programmes, procedures, and therapeutic techniques employed neither to cure the mentally ill nor to prevent mental illness but to enable or empower patients to live a better life with their disease (Roberts, Davenport, Holloway, and Tattan, 2006a). Recovery constitutes a major break with previous forms of mental treatment. First of all, it is entirely voluntary. We may recall that the history of psychiatry is notorious for the use of forced incarceration in dungeons or at mental asylums with a view to curing the patient of his madness (Foucault, 1967). We may also recall that preventive strategies targeting the mentally ill became particularly brutal during the twentieth century, when several countries saw the use of state power to control the procreation of the feebleminded and other mentally inferior groups to protect the health and vigour of the wider population (Dikötter, 1998). Secondly, recovery relies less on strictly biomedical medicine and therapies and more on various psychosocial empowerment techniques. To recover is to enhance the quality of life not in biomedical terms but in psychosocial and economic terms, i.e. to raise the self-esteem of citizens and improve their capacity to have a reasonably normal life with a family, an education, and perhaps even a job. Our motivation for focusing on recovery as the second case of health promotion is precisely because recovery does not really seek to cure illness. It seems to us that if health promotion and its strategy of empowerment can find its way into the treatment of incurable diseases, then this kind of intervention could probably find its way into any phenomena related to the improvement of human life.

To sum up, liberal democracies have seen the emergence of a new politics of health that seeks to promote the health and vigour of individuals and populations by directly targeting their conduct. While health promotion is clearly not based on coercion, it is a form of power orchestrated and often, albeit not always, implemented by state authorities that have few if any inbuilt political limitations. It is these limitless features of health promotion that call for critical scrutiny. In order to do so, we focus on two general strategies found in many health promotion interventions, namely the individualizing technologies seeking to empower citizens with a view to enable them to live a healthier life and the environmental or socializing technologies seeking to shape the social environment, networks, and relations of citizens, again, with a view towards enabling these to adopt a healthier lifestyle.

Aims and arguments

The overall aim of this book is to provide a critical understanding of current health promotion ideas and practices unfolding in liberal democracies. By 'critical' we refer to an understanding of the ways in which various power relations, expert knowledge, and social norms structure the freedom of those subjected to health promotion interventions. Of course, many existing studies critically address the shortcomings of health promotion programmes, i.e. their frequent inability to really make people healthier. However, as we will show in the following chapter, very few studies question the moral endeavour and the political strategy of health promotion, i.e. that we should constantly try to improve the health of individuals and populations and that public authorities can do only too little in securing this.

Our critical ambition is fleshed out in three more concrete aims of an empirical, conceptual, and critical character. Firstly, we seek to expose the various relations and techniques of power, expert knowledge, and social norms that constitute contemporary health promotion. This entails specifying the uniqueness of health promotion as compared to other public health strategies. Secondly, we aim to expand and qualify the conceptual debate on and understanding of contemporary tendencies in the politics of health. This implies discussing and elaborating Michel Foucault's notion of governmentality and its link to biopower (Foucault, 1978, pp. 135–159; 2007). Finally, we aim to discuss and problematize the desirability and political-ethical implications of health promotion, i.e. the promises and the limitations or costs to the freedom of citizens, patients, communities, and other subjects invoked by health promotion.

The general argument of this book is that contemporary health promotion interventions are structuring our freedom in ways that both enable new forms of freedom and limit the space of possible freedom. The empowering ambitions and techniques of health promotion work through the freedom or self-steering capacities of individuals and communities (N. Rose, 1999). In doing so, health promotion simultaneously contributes to the development of new freedoms but also imposes a number of rather strict limitations on the kinds of freedom it regards as desirable. More precisely, we argue that health promotion is a genuinely new public health strategy. It differs fundamentally from curative strategies. It also differs from earlier forms of health prevention in that it employs forms of power that directly target the conduct of citizens.

Moreover, we argue that Foucault's concepts of biopower and governmentality are both still highly useful for understanding contemporary health promotion interventions in liberal democracies. The term biopower may assist us in grasping the way in which health promotion innovates but ultimately retains the state's concern with the biological quality of the population inhabiting its territory. While the exercise of biopower in both England and Denmark has undergone tremendous changes since its emergence in the nineteenth century, notably by its increasing dependence on the self-steering capacities of individuals and communities, the term biopower is still useful in creating a space for critically analysing the ways in which state power in liberal democracies is concerned, perhaps more than ever, with the vigour of populations. The notion of governmentality allows us to address the various political rationalities at play and, at times, in conflict over health promotion. In particular, classical liberal concerns over excessive state intervention seem to be steadily losing terrain in favour of *constructivist neoliberalism* concerned with the mobilization of the self-steering capacities of individuals and communities (Triantafillou, 2017). If the term governmentality is problematic, it is because it is often used as an explanatory term, rather than a descriptive one. To be clear, we use the general term governmentality and the (more) specific term constructivist neoliberalism not to explain the emergence and functioning of health promotion but as analytical concepts that may enable us to render visible and hopefully better understand the political rationalities informing the quest for health promotion pursued not only by the state but also by a wide range of private institutions, public health experts, and other groups.

We use the term *optimistic vitalism* to characterize the particular merger between contemporary biopower and constructivist neoliberalism. We argue that contemporary health promotion is essentially a quest to improve the vigour, quality, and even happiness of the lives of individuals and populations. Contemporary health promotion interventions are widely seen as justified regardless of whether the person is seen as perfectly healthy or is diagnosed as suffering from an incurable disease. Apparently, there is always room for improving the vigour of your life. In particular, there is always room for you to reflect on yourself, on your choices around diet and physical exercise, on your coping with eventual bodily or mental maladies, and not least on how you engage with the social relations that may affect your self-esteem and choice of lifestyle. All this may sound a bit conspiratorial, as if some external machine is secretly forcing people to think in particular ways about their health. This is definitely not our understanding of optimistic vitalism, which hinges on citizens' reflecting on themselves and choosing a particular mode of conduct in order to pursue what they find is the best way to lead a vigorous and happy life. Our point is that today these reflections and choices of conduct are restricted by social norms and political programmes that urge individuals and groups to constantly think about how they can live a more vigorous and happier life in more or less particular ways.

Throughout the twentieth century, the term vitalism has served a variety of epistemological and normative purposes. The reflections of French philosopher Henri Bergson on evolution and vitalism (Bergson, 1911) inspired some to argue for a new vitalist theory or epistemological approach to biology in order to address the complexities of organic life (Hoyningen-Huene and Wuketits, 1989), while others have proposed a vitalist-materialist ethos of life celebrating becoming and transgression of boundaries (Deleuze, 1988; Braidotti, 2002). Moreover, inspired by the biological and biomedical writings of French medical doctor and philosopher Georges Canguilhem in the 1950s and 1960s (Canguilhem, 1991, 1994), we find more cautious discussions on the ability of vitalism to prepare the way for a new ethos of life (Greco, 2008), a *pathos* of life (Osborne, 2016), and to function as a principle for criticizing the normalization of life (Sholl and De Block, 2015). All these reflections are highly interesting in that they suggest that it is possible to think about and act upon life in ways that go beyond scientific biomedicine and the norms it espouses. However, they do not shed much light on the actual political exploits of vitalism today. It has been suggested that the absence of analysis of the link between vitalism and state power may be linked to a certain a priori conception of vitalism as something that transgresses state power (Villadsen and Dean, 2012). Whatever the reason, with some notable exceptions (Mills, 2013; Villadsen and Wahlberg, 2015; Wahlberg, 2016), very little has been done to critically analyse how vitalist aspirations have informed contemporary public health interventions exercised by, or at least relayed through, the state. In sum, there is a need to grasp how vitalist thinking and norms inform the exercise of biopower today. We think that obesity control and mental recovery constitute exemplary cases of health promotion, the analysis of which will allow us to better understand the particular kind of optimistic vitalism that feeds into the political ambitions of public health authorities through their attempt to govern our lives today.

Like the proponents of vitalism, this book is driven by a certain normativity. However, our concern here is not with finding a new ethos of life but with the kinds of power exercised through health promotion and the optimistic vitalism informing it. We find health promotion to be problematic because of its grand and seemingly unlimited ambitions of promoting the health of each and all by way of mobilizing society at large. If taken to its logical conclusion, health promotion may substantially reduce the space of possible freedom for the ways in which we think about and act upon ourselves in terms of health. On the one hand, we should be careful not to exaggerate the influence of health promotion vis-à-vis other health strategies. And we should be particularly careful not to overlook the fact that health promotion does allow and even stimulates new forms of freedom, whereby patients, citizens, communities, and other subjects can govern their health in novel ways that they find desirable. On the other hand, health promotion not only generates new forms of freedom, but it also actively discourages other forms, namely any form of conduct that is regarded as risky or unhealthy. Even on its own terms, health promotion is questionable as it tends to focus rather narrowly on charging individuals and communities with the responsibility of changing lifestyle choices rather than addressing wider inequalities in education and income levels. Perhaps what is particularly disconcerting is that public authorities, medical experts, and various empowerment engineers have so few qualms about intervening so extensively and quite directly into the lives of citizens and their surroundings.

The book analyses obesity control and mental recovery in England and Denmark from the 1980s until around 2015. Why these two countries? Health promotion in England and Denmark represents diversity within sameness. On the one hand, they display some fundamental similarities. Both England and Denmark have advanced relatively far in developing new ways of governing citizens, public health services, and the institutional environment supporting health interventions. They also both face relatively large problems – compared to other European OECD countries – with so-called lifestyle diseases, such as obesity, diabetes, cardiovascular diseases, and certain forms of cancer. On the other hand, the two countries differ on some important points. England is characterized by a liberal welfare regime with a strong tradition of private measures in public health and an acute sense of the problems of excessive state intervention. Although the English health services to a great extent are state-financed, as in Denmark, they nevertheless reflect strong political concerns over excessive intervention in people's lives. Denmark, on the other hand, is widely recognized for having an advanced and more or less universal welfare regime, which is supported by a widespread domestic consensus on the desirability of comprehensive state intervention to ensure the health of the population. This diversity or difference between England and Denmark is used to show that the politics of health promotion do not imply a uniform policy package but may inform quite diverse forms of political interventions.

Overview of chapters

Chapter 1 identifies and discusses the merits and the limitations of the most influential political science and sociological analyses seeking to critically address contemporary politics of health. Firstly, it focuses on studies dealing more or less directly with health promotion, i.e. the kinds of health policies that seek to improve the health of citizens through a range of empowerment strategies and programmes. Secondly, the chapter zooms in on Foucault's analytics of power and government. We account for the critical potential and limitations of Foucault's analytics and explain how they can be used to analyse power–knowledge relations and unquestioned norms in contemporary politics of health. Finally, we account for our method in terms of the cases and data selected to study the politics of health promotion in liberal democracies.

Chapter 2 seeks to provide a solid understanding of the wider political context of health promotion in England and Denmark. The chapter first delineates the emergence of biopower in the two countries during the nineteenth century. This includes accounting for the basic rationalities, interventions, and organizational structures of the public health systems. Secondly, it accounts for the major public health reforms taking place in the two countries since the 1980s with a particular focus on the health promotion strategies and programmes employed. Finally, we show how the community (or the wider institutional environment) became a site of interventions seeking to mobilize the capacity of citizens to choose and pursue healthy lifestyles.

Chapters 3 and 4 examine obesity control in England and Denmark respectively. Both chapters first briefly delineate the historical antecedents to obesity control. We then examine how political rationalities and expert knowledge mutated in both countries from around the late 1980s to render obesity an epidemiological problem requiring systematic government intervention. This was linked to political rationalities emphasizing the potential of governing through the freedom of individuals and their environments. We then move on to account for political reforms, programmes, and technologies employed to fight obesity and promote healthy lifestyles. We examine both the individualizing interventions and techniques and the programmes seeking to mobilize communities and the institutional environment in general to make it easier for citizens to eat healthily and engage in regular physical activity.

Chapter 5 and 6 analyse how and why psychiatric patients – particularly those with chronic mental illness – in England and Denmark are urged to take charge of their mental illness with reference to the notion of rehabilitation. They shed light on techniques of psychological counselling and social assistance with particular attention given to so-called Crisis Resolution and Home Treatment. As an alternative to hospital admission, these novel techniques for engaging the patients as well as the family and community expanded rapidly in England in the early 2000s. Both chapters analyse key shifts in predominant forms of political rationalities and expert knowledge on how best to treat psychiatric patients. This includes examining how the experts involved in treating the chronically mentally ill – doctors, psychiatrists, psychologists, social workers, and nurses – depend on the problematization of the targeted patients. Finally, the chapters examine how expert knowledge and political rationalities informed political interventions (policies, programmes, and technologies) in an attempt to promote rehabilitation along with increased implementation of community-based treatment.

In the conclusion we summarize and discuss the analytical findings regarding the governing of citizens through lifestyle and rehabilitation respectively. The chapter also highlights the conceptual and critical contributions to our way of understanding, debating and governing health today. Finally, it points to the needs for further research on the politics of health promotion.

1
Critical studies of the politics of public health promotion

Over the years, public health promotion has received critical attention from a wide range of academic scholars and disciplinary approaches. Much of the critique has evolved within the medical community, in which debates have taken place over the lacking (evidence of the) efficacy of specific clinical interventions and procedures (Minkler, 1999; Jackson, Waters, and Taskforce, 2005; Brownson, Baker, Leet, Gillespie, and True, 2011), and not least the tendency of medical interventions to focus rather narrowly on individuals deemed at risk, rather than focusing on the underlying causes affecting the entire population (G. Rose, 2001). While often highly critical of the state of contemporary health promotion interventions, it is usually an internal critique that only rarely touches upon the social and political dynamics shaping public health interventions. However, public health promotion has also received attention from social science scholars that explicitly addresses the social and political norms, forces, and consequences of the contemporary quest for public health promotion.

This chapter has two overall purposes: to provide an overview of existing critical social science studies of health promotion and to outline an analytical framework that will be used in the remainder of this book. Firstly, we review and discuss the merits and the limitations of the most influential political science, political economy, and sociological analyses seeking to critically address the contemporary politics of health. Secondly, we account for the Foucauldian-inspired analytical framework used in the empirical analyses of this book. This implies accounting for existing studies in the area of public health, discussing the analytical framework's potential and limitations, and accounting for the ways in which we adopt key analytical principles and concepts from Foucault's work in order to analyse power–knowledge relations and unquestioned norms in the contemporary politics of health.

14   The politics of health promotion

Critical studies of public health politics

This section reviews and discusses the potential and limitations of three general approaches for conducting critical analysis of health promotion, namely health policy process analysis, political economy, and sociological critique. The review and discussion are limited to works that deal more or less explicitly with health promotion rather than health politics in general. That is, we are interested in social science studies critically interrogating the emphasis that contemporary health politics attributes to individual lifestyle and empowerment of citizens and communities with a view towards improving the health and vigour of populations.

Policy process analysis

The aim of health policy process analysis has been formulated like this: 'to understand past policy failures and successes and to plan for future policy implementation' (Walt et al., 2008, p. 308). This may be a rather narrow definition, as some studies argue that we also need to focus on the agenda-setting and policy-formulation stages of the health policy process (T. Oliver, 2006). At any rate, based on a range of political science and public administration theories and methodologies, these studies deal with the diverse administrative, organizational, and political dynamics shaping the formulation and implementation of health policies.

Some have lamented the limited use of explicit theories in understanding and analysing health policy processes (Breton and de Leeuw, 2011). Others have pointed to the scant attention paid to politics and power in these studies (Bambra, Fox, and Scott-Samuel, 2005). Notwithstanding these discouraging assessments, we do find policy process analyses that pay attention to the kind of power relations embedded in health policies and how those power relations impinge on the target group of these policies: namely patients and citizens at large. Some have addressed the ways in which public management reforms in the health sectors from the 1980s onwards tried, with more or less success, to break with the (medical) professional authority structures found in public health institutions and services in order to hold doctors accountable for their actions (Moran, 1999; Salter, 2007). These public management reforms have arguably changed and possibly equalized doctor–patient relationships, which are increasingly characterized as a provider–consumer relationship (Hugman, 1994).

We also find critical analyses of the policy processes revolving around health promotion. The general thrust of these studies is to point to implementation failures and – in some cases – the factors or forces leading to this failure. Conversely, only very few studies pay attention to the role that agenda-setting and policy formulation play in health promotion processes (Bryant, 2002). Curiously, it is as if policy process analysts have largely ignored the political forces and conflicts engaged in setting the health agenda and formulating health promotion policies. Instead a common argument in some of the early studies was that health promotion programmes employed so far simply do not meet their goals, i.e. the programmes employed have yet to fully empower citizens and communities and, thereby, enable them to live a healthier life (Beattie, 1991; Farrant, 1991; Parish, 1995). Accordingly, the prevalence of, for example, cardiovascular diseases and type 2 diabetes is still increasing, particularly among economically disadvantaged groups. More recently, several studies have pointed to the many difficulties in empowering not only individual citizens but also local communities, which are envisaged to work in support of health promotion (Neale, Littlejohns, Hawe, and Sutherland, 2008; Baggott, 2011, pp. 367–370, 408–412; Harting and Assema, 2011; Short, Phillips, Nugus, Dugdale, and Greenfield, 2015). Such implementation deficits or even outright failures are due to a variety of factors, such as lack of an adequate programme theory, conflicting notions of success between implementation actors, and narrow vested interests among politicians and private businesses that override local community interests and needs.

In sum, political process analysis holds a strong potential for critically addressing the agenda-setting, formulation, and implementation of health promotion policies. However, the bulk of analyses have targeted only the implementation stage. Here they have pointed to the many administrative and political barriers to effective implementation. These insights are important to our understanding of why health promotion programmes often do not deliver what they promise. However, they are not very helpful in understanding why these policies were adopted in the first place. The role of knowledge, media attention, and political interests and strategies feeding into health promotion deserve much more attention than previously given. Finally, and more generally, even if the role of knowledge, media attention, and political interests were analysed, we find it an unnecessary limitation that such analysis is almost invariably couched in terms of given actors pursuing given interests. Of course, we do find policy process approaches going beyond the traditional narrow focus on actors with given interests, but they do so by drawing on political economy, ideology, sociological, and post-structuralist studies. Thus, we now turn to these latter approaches to discuss the insights they have provided and may further contribute.

Political economy and ideology studies

This section discusses the merits of approaches that focus on the ways in which socioeconomic structures connect with the design of public health interventions and institutions to produce and/or reproduce inequality in terms of income and health.

Firstly, we may note that we find a very large literature that provides evidence of inequality in the health status of populations – both within and between states (e.g. Townsend, Davidson, and Whitehead, 1988; Fein, 1995; Leon and Walt, 2000). They are critical in the sense that they locate these inequalities in differences in income, living conditions, and material opportunities in general. Low life expectancy and high incidence of diseases, even the so-called lifestyle diseases, are regarded less as the result of the randomly distributed choice of citizens or variations in individual genetic dispositions, and more as the outcome of systematic differences in the material circumstances of individuals and groups. Accordingly, in order to effectively improve health for those most prone to diseases and having low life expectancy, states should target the poor and ultimately distribute income and resources more equally. Yet if these studies are adamant that the root cause of inequality in health is inequality in income and material means, they usually have little to say about why these resources are divided so unevenly and how that links up with the provision of medical services.

Inspired more or less directly by Marxist theory, political economy approaches have tried to answer the question of why resources are so unevenly distributed within and between states so as to produce huge health differences. In a series of works, Vicente Navarro has argued that capitalist economies systematically produce economic inequalities both within states and between (the developed and developing) states (Navarro, 1976, 2002a, 2007). While capitalism may contribute to increasing general wealth, the working classes in both developed and – in particular – in developing countries will tend to become poorer. From this follows that working classes will have to work harder, will not be able to afford proper food, and will have reduced access to medical services, ultimately causing their health to deteriorate. Others have pointed out that the organization and provision of health care in capitalist societies systematically ignores occupational and social production of health and disease (Doyal and Pennell, 1979).

Recently, political economy theory approaches have been used to question the ability of health promotion interventions to secure the health of the poor and labouring classes and thereby reduce the inequality of health conditions (e.g. Dennis, 2015). A particularly good example of this literature is *The Health of Nations: Towards a New Political Economy* (Mooney, 2012), in which Mooney analyses how power is exercised both in health-care systems and in society more generally. In doing so, Mooney reveals how too many vested interests hinder efficient and equitable policies to promote healthy populations, while too little is done to address the social determinants of health. Neoliberal ideology is here taken as the main culprit for the prevalence of poor health and (social) inequality in life expectancy despite increasing resources invested in public health interventions. Along the same lines, a study of the Canadian Active Living programme argued that the quest for health promotion and empowerment in reality worked to conceal power imbalances between government officials and the community and to justify the rapid retreat of the welfare state from social responsibility for fitness and health (Bercovitz, 1998).

While we sympathize with the general ambition of problematizing the power mechanisms at stake in health promotion, we think that the political economy and ideology approaches suffer from two interrelated problems. Firstly, they seem to assume that if only the health of all citizens was elevated to a level displayed by the wealthy segments of the population, then everything would be good. However, even if we share the concern over the poor health of many citizens, in particular those with low education and low income, then it is highly problematic to assume that every person agrees to adhere to nationally given health norms. Secondly, because political economy approaches assume that all citizens desire a high and uniform level of health, then the absence of this must be due to power relations blocking poorer groups from achieving better health outcomes. Accordingly, the political economy and ideology approach focuses only on repressive forms of power, i.e. those forms of power that thwarts citizens' desires and needs. Thereby, they not only disregard the fact that some citizens – be they poor or rich – actually prefer a so-called unhealthy lifestyle. They also neglect the indirect or soft forms of power that work through citizens freely subjecting themselves to wider norms of good health. To ignore these freedom-based forms of power is problematic, as health promotion primarily, though not exclusively, relies on just these forms of power.

Sociological critique of health promotion

Ever since Émile Durkheim's famous study of suicide (Durkheim, 1968 [1897]), the influence of modern social relations on the health of individual citizens has received attention from sociologists. Variations in the health status of a population within a given state have been attributed to differences in material conditions, positioning in predominant cultural and social structures, and to the role of biomedical knowledge and authority. Today there is a very substantial body of sociological literature – both theoretical and empirical – testifying to the importance of material and social conditions, such as income level and distribution, level of education, and access to medical services, for the level and variation of citizens' health status (e.g. Macintyre, 1986; D. Gordon, 1999; Mitchell,

Dorling, and Shaw, 2000). In line with political economy approaches, these sociological studies regard differences in material conditions and economic income as crucial in shaping the possibilities that people have for leading a healthy life.

Another strand of sociological health studies have focused on the importance of trust. Trust, or rather the lack of it, between citizens in a community or between citizens and (health) authorities may contribute to poor health (Kawachi and Kennedy, 2002; Wilkinson, 2005). In particular, the last decade or two have seen the emergence of sociological research pointing to the importance of social capital for health. While some of this literature rather uncritically endorses the building of social capital as a way to promote health, we also find sociological studies critically examining how health programmes built around the notion of social capital are saturated with power relations and at times ignore material forces crucial to health outcomes (Navarro, 2002b; Wakefield and Poland, 2005). Thus, several studies of the role of socio-psychological factors for health acknowledge that low trust or social capital in certain communities often is the result of unequal distribution of material resources. Accordingly, the strictly material and many of the socio-psychological studies are highly critical of health policies that ignore the material factors impinging on citizens' health status.

A large body of sociological literature has pointed to the importance of medical knowledge and authority in shaping the relationship between doctor and patient and, more generally, the possibilities that citizens have to lead a healthy life. Several works have emerged since the 1970s criticizing the medicalization of social phenomena and, by implication, the attempt to treat social problems with medical means (Illich, 1976; see also Clarke, Shim, Mamo, Fosket, and Fishman, 2003; Conrad, 2007). Likewise, other scholars have criticized the authority exercised by the medical profession over ordinary citizens (Trostle, 1988). A somewhat different take on medical knowledge is the attempt to understand its role in formation of subjectivity. In particular, Armstrong's *A New History of Identity: A Sociology of Medical Knowledge* provides an insightful analysis of the ways in which medical knowledge and practices have contributed to the emergence of the modern human being over the last 150 years in Western, industrialized countries (Armstrong, 2002). The book provides an important historical backdrop to the current politics of health promotion by accounting for shifting medical understandings and political strategies for dealing with illness and health.

The notion that citizens' health is shaped by material, cultural, and epistemic forces and relations has also fed into sociological studies of health promotion. A general argument has been that health promotion often fails to alleviate inequality in the health of citizens, at least if it relies narrowly on biomedical expertise (Braveman, Egerter, and Williams,

2011). In fact, health promotion based on a narrow medical approach focusing on individual behaviour may perpetuate structural (social and cultural) inequalities (Bunton, Nettleton, and Burrows, 1995; M. Kelly and Charlton, 1995). According to critical sociologists, the intake of fatty foods, alcohol, tobacco, and the lack of regular physical exercise is regarded in most health promotion programmes as risky behaviour (Frohlich, Corin, and Potvin, 2001). However, what appears to be an individual choice is really a behaviour structured by social contexts and relations that induce poor people to conduct themselves in ways that are likely to lead to poor health. Thus, it has been argued that health promotion often contributes to making the individual increasingly responsible for her or his illness, including its prevention and cure (Lindbladh, Lyttkens, Hanson, and Östergren, 1998; Beck and Beck-Gernsheim, 2002). Similarly, it may contribute to the neglect of the societal or structural causes contributing to poor health. Based on this critique, a number of academics have suggested that health promotion should be designed in ways that empower communities and enhance their capacities to take care of the health of local citizens (Minkler, 2005). This may take place not through traditional medical expertise but through various forms of health education, social work, and delegation of resources to local communities.

These sociological analyses of health politics and health promotion are highly insightful in understanding why we often see wide disparities in the health of a population within and between states. However, this strength may also be a limitation. At least, most of the studies examined above are structured around the problem of how to ensure the health of citizens, rather than asking why and with what political effects are our societies seeking to improve the health and vigour of citizens and populations? That is, whereas many sociological studies are highly critical of the intentions and outcomes of health interventions, this critique revolves around the question of whether the programmes really do contribute to improving health. In other words, they tend to take the moral desirability of the quest for health improvement for granted. By the same token, power relations and the limiting effects that the quest for health improvement has on the freedom of those who are subjected to health interventions are left unquestioned. To address this issue more head-on, we suggest turning to Foucault's analytics of power and government.

Foucauldian-inspired analyses of the politics of health

Michel Foucault's historical studies of the discourses and practices of madness (Foucault, 1967), medicine (Foucault, 1973, 2000), punishment (Foucault, 1977a), modern biopower (Foucault, 1978, pp. 133–159;

2007), and modern rationalities of state governing (Foucault, 2008) have inspired a number of analyses of the modern politics of health. As our study of obesity and recovery is strongly inspired by Michel Foucault's analytical approach, it seems proper to go through existing health politics studies that use this approach. This will help clarify our contribution to the Foucauldian-inspired analysis of health politics in general and health promotion politics in particular.

While Foucault's analytics have inspired a number of studies of contemporary health interventions, only a few of these focus on modern forms of health promotion. For example, through three editions of the book *The Body and Society* published over a 20-year period, Bryan S. Turner employs an impressive range of theoretical sources to examine diverse cultural, political, and social inscriptions and regulations of the human body (Turner, 2008). While Turner does explore phenomena like the formation of dietary regimes, he does not really deal with contemporary politics of health promotion. Moreover, the edited volume *Foucault, Health and Medicine* (Petersen and Bunton, 1997) contains a number of insightful pieces that speak closely to our analysis. In particular, the pieces presented under the heading of 'governmentality' examine the linkage between the political rationalities of public health and shifting ways of governing public health. Unfortunately, the attention paid to health promotion in these essays is rather limited, which may simply have to do with timing, i.e. the rapid growth of health promotion strategies and interventions following that book's publication (see also Lupton, 2012).

A few Foucauldian-inspired works do explicitly address health promotion. Deborah Lupton (Lupton, 1995, pp. 49–61) critically addresses many of the ways in which we are urged – if not forced – to care for our health, including community empowerment, risk management, and the mass media. However, the politics of health promotion have changed since Lupton's book was published. Moreover, while Lupton is strongly inspired by Foucault, her book tends to succumb to a rather conventional understanding of power as an instrument of repression only. In effect, it is difficult to grasp why not only politicians and health workers but also many ordinary citizens accept and perhaps even enjoy taking part in health promotion efforts. Our concern is exactly to illustrate how the power invested through health promotion interventions actually depends upon the freedom and voluntary engagement of the citizens subjected to these.

In a recent monograph Brown and Baker examine the ways in which neoliberal rationalities inform health interventions in Britain and other developed states (Brown and Baker, 2012). Their key argument is that neoliberalism has unilaterally emphasized interventions seeking to promote individual responsibility at the expense of providing health services that may treat citizens for their diseases. Thus, health interventions take place through the structured freedom of individuals. A similar argument is found in Paul Crawshaw's study of technologies of social marketing in health campaigns in England (Crawshaw, 2012). His point, too, is that the Department of Health's Change4Life campaign reflects governance through self-management. In a recent book, Christopher Mayes unravels the recent political attempts to control obesity by shaping the lifestyle of citizens (Mayes, 2016). By using Foucauldian notions of biopolitics and the dispositive, Mayes undertakes a sophisticated analysis of some of the ways in which lifestyle has emerged as a network of disparate knowledge and practices through which individuals are governed towards the security of the population's health. Still, Mayes' analysis of actual political programmes and interventions is rather limited. In particular, it does not touch at all on the ways in (local) public authorities work to spin an institutional network around (obese) citizens to induce them to choose a healthy lifestyle.

While we agree with the argument that the shaping of individual freedom plays a crucial role in contemporary public health interventions, we think there is more to the story. Firstly, current health interventions are not only about creating individuals that exercise their freedom in a responsible manner. They also depend on the establishment of an institutional environment of normative and social relations that serve to assist individuals and groups in their choice of lifestyle. Secondly, we do not find it wholly satisfactory to explain the emergence of health promotion by invoking the notion of neoliberalism alone. Neoliberalism cannot be the whole story, if for no other reason than preventive and health promoting strategies were articulated long before the advent of neoliberalism. We will return to the historical precursors to health promotion in the empirical chapters on obesity control and recovery.

The role of the institutional environment in health promotion has been addressed rather infrequently by Foucauldian-inspired scholars. An early study of the WHO's Healthy Cities programme found that the advocacy of community participation in order to improve public health was based on an indirect form of power seeking to mobilize the self-steering capacities of individuals and local neighbourhoods (Petersen, 1996). Through this programme, individuals and neighbourhoods were constructed by modernist, expert knowledge as moral agents responsible for actively assisting in health improvements. A later study of the unfolding of the Healthy Cities programme in Denmark largely reached the same conclusion, though the critical emphasis here was not on the nature of modern, expert knowledge per se but rather on the absence of political limits to the kind of interventions adopted by the Healthy Cities (Frandsen and Triantafillou, 2011). Thus, the WHO's Healthy Cities programme created a new template of totalizing interventions targeting not only the sick but in principle all members of a community or a society

22   The politics of health promotion

in order promote the health and vigour of all. Another study of the treatment of suicide among bipolar patients in Denmark has shown that treatment gradually shifted after the 1970s from a focus on controlling the innate drives of the melancholic patient by secluding him within a controlled environment, the mental asylum, to a focus on the complex constellations of multiple forces that may coalesce in certain moments to increase the likelihood of the bipolar person now living in the community outside the controlled space of the asylum (Gudmand-Høyer, 2015). Even here the ever expanding logic of health promotion is unfolding in the sense that the care provided in this extra-hospital setting consists in educating the person suffering from a bipolar condition to identify the signals increasing the likelihood of suicide and equip him with tools to seek help in these situations.

The analytical framework and method adopted in this book

The analysis of obesity control and recovery pursued in this book is strongly inspired by methodological principles found in Michel Foucault's genealogical analyses of modern forms of power. When we say inspired, it is because Foucault did not provide any theoretical or methodological template for his analyses. In fact, he was at great pains to avoid any fixed analytical standards as he found this would inhibit his ambition of understanding modern power in its many forms and effects. By implication, it makes no sense to try to make a 'Foucauldian analysis', something even Foucault strictly speaking did not do. At best, we can be inspired by his insights and above all the kind of methodological principles used in his studies. By the same token, the purpose of this section is not to provide an overview of Foucault's many analyses, concepts, and methodological strategies, which has been undertaken elsewhere (e.g. Dreyfus and Rabinow, 1982; Dean, 1994; Raffnsøe, Gudmand-Høyer, and Thaning, 2016), but rather to pick a few concepts and principles that we find useful for our analysis. This section first outlines the analytical principles and concepts we adopt from Foucault. It then moves on to account for the more concrete choices of method undertaken to carry out our analysis.

A Foucauldian-inspired analytics

If we find Foucault's analysis worthy of inspiration, it is because the aim of our analysis of obesity control and recovery is congruent with the aim of his analyses, namely to critically interrogate the limits to our thinking and actions (our freedom) produced by power–knowledge relations. Foucault's analysis seeks to provide a critique based on a very thin normativity, namely maximizing the space of freedom. Accordingly, his analyses interrogate the desirability and necessity of being governed by others in a particular way (Foucault, 1997). This critique does not imply a generalized rejection of the exercise of power, something that Foucault found naïve if not undesirable, but rather that we adopt an ethos by which we remain attentive to the actual effects and limitations imposed on our freedom. Our analysis adopts this attitude in the sense that our aim is to address how it became so obvious and morally desirable to control obesity and mental diseases like schizophrenia by way of health promotion in the sense of individual and community empowerment. While our aim is to critically address obesity control and recovery, this is not to say that we regard these political strategies as necessarily bad. In fact, we believe that both obesity control and in particular recovery hold emancipatory potential for those subjecting themselves to these political strategies Rather, the aim of our analysis is to show that the rationalities, norms, and techniques making up obesity control and mental recovery rest on very specific and quite narrow norms of citizenship and community. By addressing the kinds of power and the forms of knowledge involved in health promotion, we want to examine the kind of subjectivity they seek to promote and produce. By subjectivity, we are referring to the ethical or self-governing practices that people exercise, i.e. their actual freedom. Thus, we are interested not only in the kind of power that works through objectification and perhaps even crude force but also the kinds of power that work through the subjectivity or freedom of those regarded as obese and mentally ill. In particular, we want to illuminate the moral and political limits to the freedom of citizens.

Foucault's general methodological approaches have been dubbed – by himself – as archaeology and genealogy (Foucault, 1974, 1977b). Both are essentially historical approaches that seek to illuminate the emergence and transformations of the ways in which people are constituted as subjects through systems of knowledge and various forms of power. The key rationale of these historical accounts is to show that the ways in which we think and act today are historically contingent and, by implication, that we could very well deal with mental illness, crime, sexuality, unemployment, etc. in very different ways. Both archaeology and genealogy seek to estrange us from contemporary forms of power in order to question their desirability and their necessity. The main difference between the two approaches rests with the fact that whereas archaeology mainly focuses on what are widely regarded as scientific discourses and aims to identify the regularities of their formation and transformation, genealogy pays attention both to scientific and lay knowledge. Moreover, genealogy's aim is not to map the regularities of their transformation but rather to show how they interact strategically with the exercise of power and freedom. In brief, while archaeology has the theoretical ambition of unravelling the regularities of discursive formations, genealogy has a more normative ambition: showing how we are being governed by others and by ourselves.

The analysis of obesity control and mental recovery conducted here is loosely inspired by Foucault's archaeological and genealogical analyses. On the one hand, we do not conduct a full-fledged historical analysis of these two social and political phenomena. On the other hand, we do delineate their historical precursors in England and Denmark in order to specify the historical particularity of these two phenomena. By doing so, we hope to provide a sense of just how substantially the norms and knowledge informing the exercise of power have changed in a relatively short time span. We hope too to provide a sense of estrangement from the normative ease with which many policymakers and experts in the field are participating in the quest to make people lose weight and recover from mental illness.

In order to conduct such an analysis we pay particular attention to the various kinds of power, the forms of knowledge, and not least the interrelationship between power and knowledge that make up health promotion. We are inspired by the notion of 'regime of truth', which Foucault used to distinguish his analysis from the Marxist-inspired ideology critique fashionable in the 1970s (Foucault, 1980). The notion of regime of truth denotes the procedures, rituals, and practices by which the distinction between true and false is produced in a historically specific setting or society. The analytical value of this concept is to clear a space for exposing how, on the one hand, the production of truth about a phenomenon is enabling the exercise of power over that phenomenon. On the other hand, the notion of regime of truth suggests that the production of truth is always shaped by power or, more precisely, by historically specific norms and criteria, such as randomized controlled trials.

With regard to knowledge, the point is not to gauge its truth content but to scrutinize its performative effect: What kind of problematizations and interventions in the name of health does a particular form of knowledge enable? Thus, the aim of our analysis is neither to decide whether the medical discourses about the relationship between obesity and, for example, diabetes are really true, nor whether these kinds of empowerment schemes really benefit the health of citizens. Rather, our aim in using the notion of the regime of truth is to examine the spaces of the interventions they produce, the kind of subjectivities (forms of healthy citizens) they find desirable, and how – by what techniques – attempts are made to form these subjectivities. This approach allows us to interrogate the performative effects not only of biomedical discourse, which has already been done by several critical sociologists (see above), but also pedagogical, psychological, sociological, and even post-structuralist discourses, such as those offered by Foucault (Vucina and Triantafillou,

2009). Thus, one of the analytical advantages of the notion of the regime of truth is its reflexivity. For some reason, most critical sociologists targeting the role of expert knowledge seem to focus rather unilaterally on the (repressive) effect of biomedicine but ignore the role that other scientific discourses or expert knowledges play. This limitation is particularly problematic in the case of health promotion, where not only biomedical but also pedagogical, psychological, and even sociological expertise informs the concrete debates and interventions.

Another useful concept is that of 'biopower', a term used by Foucault to denote the kind of modern power a state exercises over its population with a view to improving the latter's health and vigour (Foucault, 1978, pp. 133–159; 2007). More precisely, it points to the more or less systematic attempt to regulate disease incidence, birth rates, life expectancy, and the vigour and productivity of the population. Foucault locates the emergence of biopower in early-nineteenth-century Western Europe, when territorial states began to be increasingly concerned with the wellbeing and health of their populations. This concern was enabled by the emerging biomedical forms of knowledge, such as epidemiology, urban hygiene, social medicine, and (later) eugenics. Rather than exercising the right to take life and let live, as had been the prerogative of sovereign power, biopower is concerned with augmenting the quality and productivity of life, i.e. to create healthy and productive populations.

This conception of biopower may seem of a bit out of date today, when the concern and responsibility for public welfare is no longer only or even primarily that of the state (N. Rose, 2006, p. 63). Such concerns and responsibilities seem to be dispersed among a wide range of public and private institutions. As shown above, much of the sociological critique of contemporary health politics revolves exactly around the withdrawal of the state from the responsibility of public health and delegation of this responsibility to commercial enterprises and individual citizens. Yet we should be careful not to assume that power exercised through the state – with all the coercive potentials this implies – is obsolete in the area of health politics, including health promotion. As noted by Kaspar Villadsen and Mitchell Dean, there seems to be a certain tendency within parts of the Foucauldian-inspired governmentality studies to neglect the role of state power in the area of health and, perhaps, even celebrate vitalist norms of continuous self-creation (Villadsen and Dean, 2012). As we will show both in the Danish and English cases, the state still plays an absolutely crucial role in designing, orchestrating, and funding health promotion interventions, even if the latter seek to enable citizens and communities to care for themselves and their health. As norms of continuous self-creation and self-perfection seem to play an important role in such state interventions, we should critically interrogate what and how such norms underpin the exercise of power, not celebrate them.

Moreover, we will show that health promotion was enabled by epidemiological knowledge addressing the threats to the quality of the entire state population. Accordingly, while individuals, communities, and private companies are envisaged to play an important role in health promotion, they would not do so without the biomedical knowledge and state-orchestrated interventions targeting the population at large.

Finally, we find the term 'governmentality' useful for the purposes of this book in order to better grasp the political logics or rationalities that inform health promotion and the urge to exercise power through the self-steering capacities or freedoms of individuals and communities. This neologism (governmentality), which may be regarded as a merger of either mentality and government or rationality and government, has been used by Foucault and many after him to point to the more or less systematic secular reflections on how best to govern the security and wealth of a territorial state (Dean, 1999; Foucault, 2007). This is a highly generic term encapsulating a wide range of modern forms of state reflections, such as *raison d'état, cameralism, polizeiwissenschaft*, classical liberalism, social welfarism, and various forms of neoliberalism. If governmentality is used in a very generic fashion, the notion of 'government' was used somewhat more exclusively by Foucault to signify the kinds power that more or less systematically function by latching on to and actively facilitating the freedom of those whose conduct it seeks to shape. Government of others is a form of power that depends on the ability of those others to govern themselves. More precisely, Foucault defines government as the conduct of conduct, i.e. as the art of conducting the ways in which others conduct themselves within a more or less open field of possibilities (Foucault, 1982, pp. 220–221). As a minimum this implies that government can be exercised only over subjects that are free, i.e. who have a certain amount of room for manoeuvre in governing themselves. Yet government may go even further and more or less systematically address the possibilities of latching on to and stimulating particular forms of freedom. Foucault and others after him have thus argued that liberal government, in various ways, has hinged on the propagation and nurturing of various forms of freedom in order to govern in what it takes to be an efficient and just manner (N. Rose, 1999; Foucault, 2008).

While governing through freedom is the defining feature of liberal governmentalities, we may want to distinguish between liberalisms. Foucault made a broad distinction between classical liberalism, emerging in late eighteenth-century Britain, and neoliberalism, emerging in the US and Western Europe in the second half of the twentieth century. Like *cameralism* and *polizeiwissenschaft*, the political economy thinking formulated by Adam Smith and Adam Ferguson was concerned with the augmentation of the wealth of territorial states and the well-being of their populations. However, unlike these governmentalities, political economy, which formed the epistemic underpinning of classical liberalism, was convinced that the answer did not lie with more or less comprehensive state interventions (Foucault, 2008, pp. 1–73). Such interventions required a detailed knowledge of what the Scottish moral philosophers came to label 'civil society', i.e. all the commercial and mundane civil activities taking place between the inhabitants of a state territory. Not only would it be impossible for any institution to gain such knowledge necessary to govern correctly, the liberalists argued, it would be undesirable, because the state would inevitably debilitate the self-steering powers of civil society in its attempt to regulate it. Smith's so-called invisible hand would mean that if the state allowed citizens to pursue their own self-interest, this would augment national wealth. The role of the state should primarily be one of ensuring property, the possibility of trade and production, and upholding general law and order. In sum, classical liberal rationality of government emerges, on the one hand, as a critique of government in general and the danger of governing too much. On the other hand, it creates a new domain of governmental intervention, civil society, the self-steering capacity of which should be not only protected but also secured by the state.

Since the end of World War II, North America and Western Europe have seen the emergence of new forms of liberalism that break importantly with classical liberalism. If the defining feature of classical liberalism is protecting the self-governing capacities of citizens and civil society at large from the debilitating effects of excessive state intervention, the defining feature of neoliberalism may be elevating the market to the normative benchmark of all social activities, including those of the state. By implication, the interventions launched in the name of liberalism are concerned not so much with intruding into civil society but with enabling or even construing the conditions allowing markets to function properly. However, neoliberalism has developed in at least two quite distinct forms. Foucault identified both a US strand (Chicago School monetarism and human capital) and a West German strand (the *Ordo-Liberalen*) of advanced liberalism (Foucault, 2008, pp. 101–265). Both emerged out of a concern over (Keynesian-inspired) economic interventionism, the expansion of government administration, bureaucracy, and administration (Foucault, 2008, p. 323). However, whereas American neoliberalism tried to extend the rationality of the market and *homo oeconomicus* to all societal spheres and used this as a criterion for evaluating the suitability of the governing of health, unemployment, education, crime, etc., German neoliberalism entailed that the functioning of a rational economy required not direct state intervention but the development and maintaining of supportive conditions, regulations, and institutions. This would include not only technical, legal, and to a certain extent also financial support for economic development, but also unemployment schemes, health care systems, housing policies, etc. Neoliberal rationalities of government very similar to the German one emerged subsequently in France and a range of other (continental) Western European countries during the 1980s onwards.

Elsewhere, one of the authors of this book has used the terms *critical neoliberalism* and *constructivist neoliberalism* (Triantafillou, 2017). These terms distinguish between the forms of government informed by a critique of the state and its inability to ever get to know the true preferences of the population and the forms of government informed by the problem of how best to spur the self-steering capacities of individuals, organizations, and communities. The point is that constructivist neoliberalism does not imply a celebration of the market or a laissez-faire style of rule by which individuals are charged with the responsibility for their health situation. Rather, it implies that the state and other public authorities systematically employ their financial resources and legal powers to mobilize the self-steering capacities of individuals, communities, and organizations with a view towards bringing about politically desirable goals. These may include increasing longevity, lowering rates of diseases, and, more generally, fostering a healthy and productive population that can participate in the labour market for as long as possible. It is our contention that this constructivist neoliberalism is fundamentally informing current health interventions launched both in England and in Denmark.

Choices regarding method

We have chosen to focus on obesity control and recovery, because each represents a key case of the current quest for health promotion by way of empowering individuals and communities to take better care of themselves. The two cases are very different. Whereas obesity control is about governing a somatic phenomenon that may lead to other somatic diseases, recovery is a form of intervention addressing various mental diseases, often ones that are regarded as incurable, notably schizophrenia. Obesity control reflects what we regard as a novel and controversial element of health promotion, namely the attempt to ensure the health of the population by targeting individuals who are currently not regarded as sick – at least not according to contemporary medical science. The proliferation of the notion of risk in the politics of health implies that all are potential targets of health interventions. Thus, contemporary health promotion works under the assumption that we are all at risk of becoming ill and that everyone can improve his or her behaviour in order to minimize that risk.

In contrast, recovery reflects just how strongly current health politics believes in the virtues of empowering individuals and communities. One could assume that the quest for constantly improving the productivity and vigour of people would at least not apply to those deemed incurably ill, an understanding that has prevailed until recently in the case of schizophrenia. Not so anymore. Presently, schizophrenic patients are subjected to mental recovery even if the chances of curing them (in the sense of removing their clinical symptoms) are meagre. It seems to us that if the notion of empowerment can find its way into the care of diseases that are widely regarded as very difficult – if not outright impossible – to cure, such as schizophrenia, then it could probably find its way into any medical phenomena. In fact, a recent Danish study of the treatment of bipolar condition shows just this (Gudmand-Høyer, 2015). While the two cases certainly are not representative of the manifold and variegated interventions seeking to promote health, their very extremity may be useful to understand how and why, the current quest for health promotion emerged and with what political and ethical effects.

The temporal focus of our analysis lies with the period from the 1990s until 2015. This is the period when the present strategies and programmes of health promotion grew rapidly, starting with the WHO's Health for All strategy launched in the late 1980s. While we go into some detail about the reforms taking place in Denmark and England in that period, we are not trying to map out all the interventions that may have something to do with health promotion. Rather we are focusing on major political reforms linked to health promotion on the one hand, and zoom in on the more specific interventions and institutions employed in obesity control and recovery on the other.

While our temporal focus is on the events taking place since the 1990s, we also make a brief account of preventive health interventions taking place in the 1920s and 1930s under the heading of eugenics in Denmark and England. While clearly not fully fledged genealogical analyses as explained above, the purpose of this brief historical backdrop is similarly to expose the specificity of contemporary health promotion. On the one hand, the eugenics movement and interventions of the interwar period display several similarities with current health promotion in their strong emphasis on preventive strategies. By implication, like current health promotion, the eugenics movement was not only targeting the sick but was also about targeting the entire population of the state in order to improve its health and vigour. At the same time, there are several fundamental differences between the interwar eugenics movement and current health promotion, the most fundamental being the crucial role attributed to individual and community empowerment since the 1990s.

We chose Denmark and England because their pursuit of public health and welfare are usually regarded as being underpinned by very different political ideologies or, as we prefer, political rationalities. Denmark is seen as one of the leading exponents of social welfarism, in which solidarity and social insurance is employed to provide universal access to welfare goods. In contrast, England is regarded as one of the leading exponents of liberalism, whereby the goal of public welfare and health is carefully balanced – if not overshadowed – by concerns for individual liberty, concerns over excessive state intervention, and a strong emphasis on individual responsibility. In such different political ideological climates, it is particularly interesting to see how health promotion plays out. We pay attention to both the differences and the similarities in the ways in which the two countries pursue obesity control and mental recovery.

Of course, the differences between the political systems in Denmark and England should not be exaggerated. Both countries are economically advanced and prosperous, with firmly entrenched traditions of liberal democracy. Moreover, the health system in both countries is entirely tax-funded, strongly regulated by central government, and largely provided by public institutions. Thus, both health systems fit the national health service model (Blank and Burau, 2014, pp. 11–13). Within this broad similarity of the health systems, we find some important differences: the English is an integrated national one, the National Health Service; the Danish system is divided between the regions, responsible for hospital services, and the municipalities, which are in charge of preventive and rehabilitative interventions. We thus pay attention to whether this organizational difference may matter for the employment of health promotion programmes in the two countries.

Finally, regarding collection of data, we rely almost exclusively on publicly available documents. Two general types of documents have been collected: public health policy documents published by various public authorities in Denmark and England, and expert documents issued by doctors, psychiatrists, psychologists, social workers, economists, sociologists, and political scientists, which provide analyses and recommendations on how to design and improve ongoing health promotion efforts. The health policy documents from Denmark were collected by going through the homepages of the Danish Health Authority, Danish Regions, and Local Government Denmark. We used the reference lists of these documents to locate other relevant documents. We also made searches in the national database bibliotek.dk and simple searches in google.dk with the terms: 'sundhedsfremme', 'forebyggelse', 'overvægt', 'fedme', and 'recovery'. In England, the homepages of the National Health Service and the Local Government Association were searched for documents dealing with health promotion, prevention, obesity, recovery, and community participation. Again, the reference lists of the documents here were used to identify other relevant documents. Finally, we made google.com searches using the terms 'England', 'health promotion', 'prevention', 'obesity', and 'mental recovery'.

With regard to expert documents, we searched Web of Science (social science citation index) and Scopus using the terms 'health promotion', 'prevention', 'obesity', 'recovery', and 'community participation'. We did not go through the biomedical databases, as a quick search there indicated that we would have to go through a very large volume of mainly irrelevant articles focusing narrowly on the biomedical/clinical aspects of obesity and mental recovery. As our aim was not to map the breadth of biomedical knowledge on obesity and recovery but instead how this knowledge more or less directly informed health politics, we carefully went through the references in the policy documents mentioned above to see what kind of expert discourses (medical and non-medical) they were drawing on. We then collected these expert publications and analysed their way of problematizing and objectifying the issues of obesity and recovery and unravelled the kind of interventions they proposed.

Finally, it may be worth briefly justifying the absence of other types of data. Why not, for example, conduct interviews with policymakers, frontline workers, or citizens engaged in health promotion? In strictly analytical terms, the reason for this absence is that the aim of our analysis is to unravel the problematizations, rationalities, programmes, and techniques employed in obesity control and recovery. These can all be accounted for by the use of documents. The goal of our analysis is neither to unravel the political compromises behind public health interventions (taking place behind closed doors) nor to understand the motivation of the target groups for participating or not in obesity control or recovery programmes. This being said, we do agree that interviews with frontline workers and citizens could have provided a richer account of the concrete ways in which the interventions were employed, including the ways in which the procedures and techniques for empowering citizens and communities were brought into play. We partly cover this dimension in the Danish case by drawing on a hitherto unpublished PhD dissertation about health promotion in Denmark (Vucina, 2014). In the English case, we occasionally draw on interviews given within existing studies when we find that these may illustrate the particular functioning of a concrete intervention in the area of obesity control or recovery.

Conclusion

This chapter has provided an overview of existing critical social science studies of health promotion and outlined an analytical framework that will be used in the remainder of the book. The review showed that we find a number of critical social science studies of contemporary politics of health, including health promotion. We found four approaches particularly influential in the field: political science-inspired policy process analysis, political economy approaches, sociological analyses, and Foucauldian-inspired works. We argued that all four approaches have strong critical potential. Yet for our purposes, the Foucauldian-inspired framework seems the most viable one. The main reason for this is its reflexive capacity or, put differently, its explicit targeting of the ways in which all kinds of expert knowledge, including Foucauldian analysis itself, may inform the exercise of power. Thus, it opens up for analysis the role played not only by biomedical expertise but also a range of pedagogical, psychological, sociological, and even post-structuralist knowledge in the pursuit of health promotion.

Accordingly, we accounted for the Foucauldian-inspired analytical framework used in the empirical analyses of this book. Instead of trying to account for the entirety of Foucault's analyses and concepts, we adopted a few analytical principles and key concepts found to be particularly relevant for our purposes. We accounted for key terms like biopower, governmentality, and neoliberal government, which will be used in subsequent analysis. Finally, we provided some reflections on our method, including choice of cases (country and disease types) and data.

2

Governing public health in England and Denmark

The aim of this chapter is to provide a solid understanding of the historical and political contexts of the obesity and recovery-orientated interventions analysed in the proceeding chapter. The wider purpose of this historical and political contextualization is to get a better insight into the ways in which health promotion is unfolding in England and Denmark. This implies grasping both the essential differences and the many similarities. Accordingly, this chapter looks at both the similarities and the main differences between the key historical reforms and approaches in the governing of health in England and Denmark.

We argue that three general strategies for the governing of health can be found in both countries: prevention, cure, and promotion. These are distinct but interrelated strategies. All three strategies are still important today, though health promotion has come to play a hitherto unseen important role in Danish and English health policies since around 1990. Another key argument is that, while we do find important differences between Danish and English health politics in terms of administrative setups, the relative importance of liberal rationalities of government, and the role played by the community in health promotion, we also find profound similarities both in terms of the overall importance attributed to health promotion and in terms of the various types of programmes and techniques employed to empower citizens and communities in the name of health.

The chapter starts out by delineating the historical emergence of biopolitics from the nineteenth century in the two countries. This section is relatively brief but essential to identify key reforms, approaches, and the administrative organization of the governing of health still persisting today in the two countries. The chapter then moves on to the 1980s to explore the turn towards health promotion and to discuss its wider implications for biopolitics in the two countries. Finally, the chapter examines how the community has been invoked in both countries, albeit in different ways, in the attempt to promote the health of citizens.

The emergence of biopolitics in England and Denmark

This section delineates the historical emergence and key features of biopolitics from the nineteenth century in the two countries. More precisely, we illuminate key features of the governing of public health taking place through the public authorities in England and Denmark. This entails identifying major reforms, approaches, and the administrative organization of the governing of health, features that to a large extent persist today in the two countries. Conversely, the intention is not to provide a comprehensive account of all the manifold public health ideas and reforms that have taken place in England and Denmark.

England

Until around the mid-nineteenth century few would have predicted that Britain would, in a few decades, have developed a comprehensive and intrusive public health apparatus. Until then the state's health interventions had mainly functioned through the Poor Laws, dating back to the sixteenth century (Dean, 1991). While the development of the correction house system in the early seventeenth century implied comprehensive and often forced intervention into the lives of paupers, there was nothing to suggest or legitimize state interventions in the lives of the working classes or the wealthy. In fact, the liberal rationalities of government prevailing from the end of the eighteenth century would make such interventions appear illegitimate and unlikely.

This would all change during the nineteenth century. With the growth of industrialization and large-scale urbanization, England saw an explosion of workers living under miserable conditions. Not only were infant death rates very high; adults succumbed to epidemics, such as cholera, scarlet fever, smallpox, and typhus. All these diseases thrived in the densely populated and unhygienic urban centres. Liberal concerns over the dangers and futility of state intervention notwithstanding, the emergence of health and social statistics (epidemiology), which rendered mortality and sickness visible on a national level, combined with the development of influential voices arguing for the need of public health interventions, paved the way for the Public Health Acts of 1848 and 1875. Worried that they too would suffer from the diseases flourishing among workers and paupers, the rising capitalist bourgeoisie was concerned over the productivity of labour power, and state officials were increasingly convinced that raising the general health of the population was necessary to ensure the development of national wealth (Leichter, 1991, pp. 36–37).

During the nineteenth century, the state would develop and pursue a politics of health that, crudely speaking, evolved around two poles: *prevention* via modification of the physical environment and *curation* via the supply of medical services available to most citizens (Brend, 1917). The immediate aim of the 1848 Public Health Act was to spur the construction of water supply and sewage systems in order to prevent the spread of infectious diseases, such as cholera. While the Pasteurian bacterial revolution did not occur until the end of the century, miasmic theories of the negative impact of foul air, odours, and filth drove several comprehensive reforms seeking to improve the miserable and unhygienic living conditions in the growing urban centres (Ackerknecht, 1968, pp. 210–217). This is also the period that saw the general vaccination against smallpox – starting with children in 1840. The next half-century would see an unprecedented development of state interventions in the name of curing illness and securing the health of the population. The Public Health Act's regulation of urban water supply and sewage systems was followed by the 1858 Medical Act, which allowed the state to regulate the provision of medical services by doctors, who had to be licensed and included into a single national register.

There is little doubt that modifications of the physical environment, with a view towards improving hygienic conditions, constituted the predominant form of preventive health strategy in Britain in the first half of the twentieth century (McKeown, 1979). However, two other preventive strategies played a significant role in early British health policy: inoculation and eugenics. Introduced in 1840 as a voluntary measure, inoculation against smallpox was made compulsory for all infants in 1853 and for all under the age 14 in 1867. Although forced inoculation was met with substantial resistance from various political, scientific, and Christian groups (MacLeod, 1967a, 1967b), the new biopolitical ambition seemed to legitimize coercive state interventions. Eugenics is worth mentioning, too, even if its impact never really moved from the level of scientific ideas to political action. The British eugenics movement was particularly influential around the turn of the century, when the urban crisis of the 1880s and the Boer War of the 1890s provided fertile grounds for ideas about negative eugenics (MacKenzie, 1976). With Francis Galton and Karl Pearson as leading proponents, the Eugenics Education Society was established in 1907 to promote public understanding about eugenics and to propagate birth-control regulations. In that period the movement received support from many politicians of both conservative and socialist orientations. A number of social hygiene organizations continued to discuss and argue for the need to control the procreation of the unfit and improve the quality and efficiency of the working class during the interwar period (G. Jones, 1986). Attempts to authorize forced sterilization in Britain peaked during the debates over the Mental

Deficiency Acts in 1913 and 1927, and a special committee (the Brock Committee) was formed under the Ministry of Health in 1932 to draw up a programme for sterilization of the feeble-minded in England and Wales (King, 1999, pp. 64–80). However, all these attempts failed due to resistance from liberal politicians, parts of the labour movement, critical scientists (the British Medical Association), and not least the Christian clergy. Thus, even if the procreation of the feeble-minded and the morally depraved did constitute a concern in England during the first half of the twentieth century, this did not lead to forced sterilization as was the case in the Nordic countries, Germany, and parts of the US (Thomson, 1998). Moreover, while members of the Eugenics Education Society tried to revive political attention to the need for controlling the procreation of the feeble-minded after the end of World War II, this attempt remained unsuccessful, partly due to changing medical understandings of mental deficiency, which entailed an increased confidence in the potential of correct child rearing and therapeutic treatment (G. Jones, 1986, pp. 148, 152–153).

In addition to the aforementioned preventive approach, a systematic curative approach was developed simultaneously through shifting British governments' support of the establishment of more public hospitals and infirmaries intended for the poor and improving the standard of medical services at these institutions (Ham, 2009, pp. 7–11). The development of modern hospital services catering for the sick was spurred by the 1867 Metropolitan Poor Act, which applied to London, and was soon followed by the development of public hospital services in other urban areas. This curative approach was further consolidated during the first half of the twentieth century. In 1911, the National Insurance Act was adopted in order to expand popular access to medical services by providing free care by GPs for certain groups of low-paid working people, and in 1948 the National Health Service (NHS) was established in order to coordinate the development of hospitals and their services and to extend health insurance to more groups (Ham, 2009, pp. 13–14). The new service entailed that both local (public) and voluntary (private) hospitals were placed under one single system of administration, that all citizens were covered by health insurance, and that the health services were mainly funded out of general taxation – rather than individual insurance contributions.

The establishment of the NHS may be taken as an indication of just how far social welfarist rationalities had come to prevail over the former classical liberal ones. Yet one should be careful to understand the role these rationalities played in British health politics during the nineteenth and the first half of the twentieth century. The public health interventions employed through the state apparatus were comprehensive and aspired to ensure the health of all citizens. However, neither of these approaches directly targeted the everyday conduct of individuals.

Moreover, with inoculation as an important exception, British health politics did not employ coercion. Instead, the biopolitical interventions evolved around prevention working through modifying the physical environment and around the provision of curative services. These strategies fit relatively well with liberal concerns over excessive state intervention (Osborne, 1997).

Denmark

As in England, the Danish state's concern over the health and vigour of its population gained momentum around the mid-nineteenth century. The turn towards a modern biopolitics came with the cholera outbreak in Copenhagen in 1853 and other Danish cities in the same decade. The growth of epidemiological data tracing the incidence of cholera by place and time was used to suggest all kinds of correlations between cholera on the one hand, and weather conditions, the day of the week, gender, and, fortunately, also living conditions on the other (Larsen, 2014, pp. 124–130, 157–162). Together with miasmic theories, these statistics informed the work of several health commissions, which recommended the supply of clean drinking water, urban sewage and garbage collection systems, new urban design principles and housing standards, the hygienic handling of food, and various inoculation campaigns. Notwithstanding resistance from conservative politicians and private real estate owners, most of these proposals were translated into political reforms that changed the physical appearance of Copenhagen and other major urban areas quite radically during the late nineteenth century. For example, the ban on settlements outside the medieval part of Copenhagen in order to ensure the defence of the city in case of an attack was abandoned in the early 1860s and followed by rapid expansion of the city (Lützen, 1998). Co-operative (self-owned) housing associations were formed – often with public support – to build healthy and hygienic apartments at affordable prices to workers and other groups with relatively low incomes. Also, public parks and swimming facilities were established to allow urban dwellers access to light, fresh air, and occasional exercise.

As in England, inoculation and eugenics play a limited but not insignificant role in the biopolitical endeavour developing from the early nineteenth century. A state regulation was adopted in 1810 whereby any person who wanted to be baptized, to be married, or to enter schools or the military had to be inoculated against smallpox (*Forordning om koppevaccination 1810*, 2016). The law was later expanded to include all citizens and was only abandoned in 1976 – following six years with no new outbreaks. However, the law on smallpox inoculation is unique in Danish health policy in that no other inoculations were mandatory. As in

England, heated scientific and political debates took place over eugenics and birth control in the interwar period. Unlike the case in England, these debates were translated into political action, notably the adoption of three laws in the late 1930s enabling sterilization of the feeble-minded, the mentally ill, and sexual criminals, termination of pregnancy among feeble-minded women, and the prohibition of marriage between feeble-minded persons (Koch, 1996). Informed by hereditary theories and the developing welfare economics, as articulated famously by the Swedish couple Alva and Gunnar Myrdal, the overriding argument for these laws was that the only way to secure the quality of the population and to build an economically viable welfare state was to hinder the unproductive classes from procreating (Koch, 1996, pp. 174–175). Even if forced sterilization was only applied in the case of sexual offenders, the following three decades saw the sterilization of several thousand persons regarded as feeble-minded, mostly alcoholics and prostitutes from the lower classes.

With the concern for the population's health came the establishment of new hospitals and reformation of existing ones. Several hospitals had been established by the state and other public authorities already during the mid-eighteenth century (Vallgårda, 1989). However, at that time, the hospitals mainly served to assist the poor and to prevent the spread of disease. During the nineteenth century the poor were evicted from the hospitals, which were now turned exclusively into sites for the treatment of the sick (Larsen, 2014, pp. 210–216). In order to expand the availability of curative services to the Danish population, a reform was adopted in 1892 that gave public support to existing private health insurance associations. These associations had previously been directly linked to the guilds and craft associations, and from around the mid-nineteenth century they had usually received modest and uneven levels of municipal support. With the Law of Authorized Health Insurance Associations of 1892, the government supported the expansion of health insurance coverage of workers and farmers and effectively gave most citizens access to both (private) general practitioners and to the increasing number of public hospitals (Jonasen, 2003, pp. 104–105).

In brief, modern biopolitics emerged in Denmark around the mid-nineteenth century and evolved around both prevention and curative approaches. As in England, modifications to the physical environment to improve hygiene constituted the key preventive strategy. However, a major difference between the two countries is that in Denmark negative eugenics were translated into quite comprehensive interventions. As in England, the state and other public authorities invested heavily in making medical services widely available and affordable through general practitioners and public hospitals. Danish public health policies were informed by a mix of social welfarist and liberal rationalities of government. They were social welfarist in so much as they aimed at socializing the costs of health services – first through privately designed social insurance mechanisms and later by a system financed through taxation. However, they were also liberal in that they mainly focused on curative strategies and usually had no ambitions to intervene in the conduct of individuals. Perhaps this mix was conducive to an atmosphere of political consensus around public health policies that prevailed throughout the twentieth century. Debates over the size of the public health budgets and regulation of the medical profession notwithstanding, liberal, conservative, and social democratic parties have tended to agree on the importance of providing extensive publicly financed health services to the Danish people. On the one hand, then, the Danish politics of health display strong similarities to those of England in terms of the health intervention approaches and rationalities informing these. On the other hand, the two countries differ importantly regarding the actual engagement in sterilization of the feeble-minded in the mid-twentieth century in order to ensure the welfare state's economic sustainability.

The turn towards health promotion

This section examines the turn towards health promotion in England and Denmark from around the 1980s. It discusses how the advent of health promotion recast existing biopolitics. Both the English and the Danish turn towards health promotion was explicitly inspired by the WHO's new Health for All by the Year 2000 strategy, which was launched in the mid-1980s. In 1984 the WHO's European Region adopted targets on Health for All (WHO Regional Office for Europe, 1985). The targets were part of a strategy for ensuring '[h]ealth for all by the year 2000'. This strategy recommended that states ensure the development of a comprehensive set of basic support functions within a wide array of societal sectors in order to promote a healthy lifestyle, healthy environment, and an adequate health service. Improving public health meant changing lifestyle. The latter was regarded as not only an individual matter but also as something requiring comprehensive interventions by public authorities. Two years later the WHO explicated this new strategy in its Ottawa Charter:

> [H]ealth promotion demands coordinated action by all concerned: by governments, by health and other social and economic sectors, by nongovernmental and voluntary organizations, by industry and by the media ... Health promotion goes beyond health care. It puts health on the agenda of policy makers in all sectors and at all levels, directing them to be aware of the health consequences of their decisions and to accept their responsibilities for health ... Health promotion policy

> requires the identification of obstacles to the adoption of healthy public policies in non-health sectors and ways of removing them. The aim must be to make the healthy choice the easier choice for policy makers as well. (World Health Organization, 1986, p. 2)

The WHO's new health promotion strategy came along with a number of targets for health improvements. However, the strategy's defining feature was not its targets or its vaguely formulated instruments to reach them but rather its strategy and the rationality informing it. Health promotion entailed the continued improvement of health for all – not just the ill – and in order to pursue this end all parts of society had to be mobilized. Central to this approach has been an intense debate that health promotion has not been sufficiently devoted to strengthen health, but retained a focus on diseases and their prevention (e.g. Antonovsky, 1996). This debate suggests that the new health promotion approach has hardly replaced, but rather supplemented and ultimately recast, existing curative and preventive strategies. Over the next decade or so, health promotion would be politically endorsed in both England and Denmark, though this endorsement cannot be attributed only to the WHO. As we will show, a number of national developments, notably the rapidly increasing number of lifestyle diseases and the development of wider neoliberal rationalities in both countries, would contribute importantly to the spread and consolidation of health promotion.

England

The understanding that illness and poor health result not only from poor physical conditions or the absence of health services, but also – and more importantly – from individual attitudes and behaviours emerged in England (and other parts of Britain) at the end of the 1970s (Leichter, 1991, p. 76). A report made on the initiative of the House of Commons to examine the causes of the increasing costs of the NHS concluded that much of this expense was due to undesirable individual behaviour and that more emphasis should be placed on prevention (Leichter, 1991, p. 79). This report was followed by a White Paper issued by the Labour government, *Prevention and Health*, which acknowledged that '[t]oday, the greatest scope for further progress [in public health] would seem to lie in seeking to modify attitudes and behaviour in relation to health' (Department of Health and Social Security, 1977, p. 10). This understanding would gradually gather pace during the 1980s in a political thought space increasingly informed by the neoliberal rationalities espoused by the Thatcher government (Leichter, 1991, p. 90).

Yet the importance ascribed to the individual choice of lifestyle for public health did not immediately translate into political action. At least, changing British governments were not inclined to launch interventions directly targeting citizens' lifestyle. For example, until the 1990s, attempts to reduce smoking mainly relied on voluntary agreements with the tobacco industry for warning labels on cigarette packages and curbing cigarette advertisements (Leichter, 1991, pp. 126–127). Liberal rationalities prevailed even more strongly in the (lack of) regulation of alcohol consumption in the same period, despite the fact that it was widely recognized as both a medical and social problem (Leichter, 1991, pp. 179–180). This reluctance to engage in preventive health strategies was due to a combination of liberal concerns over infringement of individual liberty, individual victimization, and the absence of clear scientific support for the effectiveness of health prevention interventions (Leichter, 1991, pp. 80–83).

Health promotion strategies only emerge from the early 1990s, taking inspiration from the WHO's strategy Health for All by the Year 2000. The WHO strategy emphasized the need not only for preventive but also health promotion strategies (World Health Organization, 1986).[1] In 1992, the Conservative government published the White Paper *The Health of the Nation – A Strategy for England*, which outlined a comprehensive strategy for improving the entire population's health (Secretary of State for Health, 1992). The new British strategy aimed not only at reducing illness but also at promoting health. This is how the Secretary of State for Health, Virginia Bottomley, explained the new health strategy:

> There was support [in the debate following the Green Paper 'The Health of the Nation', 1991] for the need to concentrate on health promotion as much as health care; for the need to set clear and challenging targets – and not too many of them – at which to aim; and for the need for all of us to work together. (Secretary of State for Health, 1992, p. 2)

Apart from the WHO's strategy Health for All by the Year 2000, the English Health of the Nation strategy was informed by recent epidemiological studies of the British population's major diseases, life expectancy, etc. Together they led to the identification of five priority areas of intervention, namely coronary diseases, cancer, mental illness, HIV/AIDS and sexual health, and accidents. In order to reach the targets set for these five areas, the strategy implied concerted efforts by a wide array of actors, central and local, public and private, such as the NHS, the Department of Environment, the Health Education Authority, local authorities, voluntary organizations, the media, schools, and workplaces (Secretary of State for Health, 1992, pp. 23–25). While the Secretary of State does point out in the White Paper's Introduction that 'families and individuals themselves must contribute if the strategy is to succeed' (Secretary of State for Health, 1992, p. 3), the remainder of the White Paper focuses exclusively on the role of various inter-sectoral programmes assisting behavioural change, such as making citizens adopt a healthier diet, reduce or stop smoking, and engage in more physical activity.

The Health of the Nation strategy is quite open about its insecurity regarding how to successfully make citizens change their behaviour in a more healthy direction through the use of only voluntary means. Over and over again, the report articulates the need for further research in this area. Until then, the strategy was bound to rely on a mixture of providing information, guidelines for action, and care services to meet the various health targets. Unsurprisingly, the impact of the new strategy on the design of health services seemed to have been quite limited, perhaps because most public health interventions taking place during the mid-1990s retained a focus on the performance of delivery of curative health services, such as cutting waiting times (Department of Health, 1998).

While its start may not have been very successful, the health promotion strategy had not been forgotten. With the White Paper *Saving Lives: Our Healthier Nation*, the New Labour government launched a concerted and preventive strategy targeting the major diseases affecting public health, such as cancer, heart diseases, mental illness, and various accidents (Secretary of State for Health, 1999a). Like its Conservative predecessor, the New Labour health strategy aimed not only at preventing and reducing these illnesses but also at building a healthier nation by improving the health of everyone. By making the British population adopt a healthier lifestyle it was imagined that it would be possible to curb growing public health expenditure (Wanless, 2004; Department of Health, 2010, p. 5). The way to make individuals adopt a healthier lifestyle, i.e. proper diet, engaging in more physical activity, and reducing smoking and alcohol consumption, was to make the NHS, communities, and families work together. This entailed, on the one hand, addressing social and environmental factors shaping the choice of lifestyle, and, on the other hand, more direct and individualizing interventions, such as online information and professional counselling on how to change one's lifestyle. These programmes were linked to a series of national targets for the improvement of the population's health, notably lower death rates incurred by major illnesses.

New Labour took its health promotion strategy a step further with its 2004 White Paper *Choosing Health: Making Healthy Choices Easier* (Department of Health, 2004). Again, citizens were to make the right choice thanks to the provision of adequate information and personalized support tailored to the individual's situation, on the one hand, and by promoting cooperation between health authorities, communities, and individuals on the other. In line with the WHO's 'whole system approach' mentioned above, the New Labour government insisted on the role of nurturing the so-called communities, private companies, and families to create an environment that makes it easier for individuals to make the right choice. Moreover, socioeconomic differences in health standards played an important role in informing the Blair government's attempts to improve public health, such as the Neighbourhood Renewal strategy. The comprehensive £75 million Change4Life programme launched in 2009 bore witness to the importance attributed by the New Labour government to the rationality of individual citizens in making the right choice of lifestyle (Baggott, 2013, pp. 112–113). Yet neighbourhood renewal, it was believed, would not come by itself but by way of a comprehensive network of efforts and actors ranging from individual exercise and diet programmes, parental training and workplace schemes to neighbourhood programmes including local schools, GPs, and others. Also instrumental to neighbourhood renewal was the work of health promotion or health improvement practitioners, including people with a degree in medicine, nursing, psychology, or social work, who had to act not only as experts within their field, but also as facilitators stimulating the inculcation of norms of healthy living among individuals and neighbourhoods alike. Accordingly, we find the claim that New Labour's emphasis on lifestyle choice entails a thoroughly individualistic approach to the governing of public health to be, if not outright wrong, then at least much too simplistic (Hunter, Marks, and Smith, 2010, p. 75).

On the face of it, the advent of the new Coalition government made up of the Conservative and Liberal Democratic parties in 2010 seemed to imply the demise of the role of the public health services in health promotion. At least, it would seem obvious that the new government would emphasize the role of individual needs and responsibilities in choosing a healthy lifestyle. While it is true that the NHS underwent significant reforms during 2010–2012 that resulted in a larger role for private actors in the provision of health services, the NHS did not see the kind of dramatic budget cuts that most other public sectors did, though this remains a contested issue (e.g. Ross, 2012). At any rate, the importance of tailoring health interventions to specific individual needs and circumstances was reiterated by the Coalition government's White Paper *Healthy Lives, Healthy People* (Department of Health, 2010). This report found that earlier efforts seeking to tackle the major public health menaces, such as obesity, smoking, drug use, sexually transmitted infections, and poor mental health and health inequality, had been ineffective because: 'it is simply not possible to promote healthier lifestyles through Whitehall diktat and nannying about the way people should live' (Department of Health, 2010, p. 2). In order to work effectively, public health interventions must instead 'empower people to make healthier choices and give communities the tools to address their own, particular needs' (Department of Health, 2010, p. 2).

Again, this may be taken to be a simple laissez-faire strategy that reduces public health policies to a question of individual choice (Corbett and Walker, 2012). But while the rhetoric of the Coalition government may have downplayed the role of the NHS and the so-called community in favour of private companies and workplaces, it still launched a series of measures to create an institutional setting conducive to making the right lifestyle choice. In a follow-up to the *Healthy Lives, Healthy People* White Paper, it was emphasized that local authorities should play a crucial role of providing targeted health services and adopting behavioural techniques that would assist citizens in making healthy lifestyle choices (Secretary of State for Health, 2011). Together with the NHS, local authorities are envisaged to engage in tobacco control, alcohol, and drug misuse services, obesity and community nutrition initiatives, and efforts to promote physical activity in the local population (Secretary of State for Health, 2011, p. 27). While the report remains conspicuously vague on how – by what concrete mechanisms and techniques – local authorities are supposed to engage in health promotion, it is clearly not simply pursuing a laissez-faire health policy. In fact, the Healthy Lives strategy is explicitly endorsing the so-called Marmot Report, *Fair Society, Healthy Lives*, which takes inequality in health as the key challenge to English health policies (The Marmot Review Team, 2010). The report, orchestrated by Professor Michael Marmot, recommended that in order to reduce health inequalities in England it is necessary to develop healthy and sustainable workplaces and communities, strengthen the role and impact of local delivery systems, promote participatory decision-making, and empower individuals and local communities. While the report had been solicited by the former New Labour Health Secretary, it did fit fairly well with the Coalition government's commitment to health promotion for everyone by way of invoking the forces of local communities and private engagement.

Apart from mobilizing local authorities and communities, the Coalition government seemed to pin great hope on the potential of behavioural change methods to make citizens adopt healthier lifestyles (R. Jones, Pyket, and Whitehead, 2013, pp. 120–121). Based on the insights of behavioural psychology, a series of techniques – often lumped together under the heading of nudging – were to be employed with a view towards modifying citizens' everyday choices. Unlike economic incentives, nudging is neither a question of appealing to the self-interest of the rational actor nor is it about raising the self-esteem of the obese. Rather, nudging seeks to manipulate the circumstances that shape our unconscious choices of conduct, such as small arrows leading to the staircase (rather than to the elevator), putting healthy food rather than sweets in front of the counter at canteens and supermarkets, and providing bike lanes rather than fast car routes. Inspired by Thaler and Sunstein's *Nudge* (Thaler and Sunstein, 2008), David Cameron inaugurated the Behavioural Insights Team (BIT), or simply the Nudge Unit, in 2010 with a view towards providing advice on how to secure better policy implementation in ways that minimized the state dictating individual choice. BIT issued the document *Applying Behavioural Insights to Health*, which argued that nudging could play an important role in making the British adopt healthier lifestyle choices, including organ donation, avoiding teenage pregnancy, reducing alcohol consumption, improving diet, and increasing physical activity (Cabinet Office, 2011). However, while the idea of nudging actually emerged some time prior to the Coalition government, there have so far been only few systematic attempts to nudge or change the choice architecture to make people make healthier choices in England. Thus, apart from prompting citizens to choose in relation to organ donation (Behavioural Insights Team, 2013), it seems that we still await centrally orchestrated attempts to employ nudges with a view towards promoting healthy lifestyles.[2] Similarly, as we will see in the next chapter, the use of nudging in obesity control remains quite limited.

In brief, the Coalition government's health promotion strategy was not just a continuation of New Labour's strategy in as much as it aimed at adopting a 'least intrusive approach' (Department of Health, 2010, p. 6). It is also true that the Coalition government and the present Conservative government have both been quite vague on just how – by what means – they envisage that local authorities and communities are supposed to promote the health of local citizens. Yet the concern with the health of the English population clearly goes beyond purely curative approaches and endorses both community-orientated interventions and various behavioural campaigns and techniques (nudging) with a view towards making individuals change their everyday conduct.

Denmark

During the 1990s, Danish health policies changed slowly but significantly by increasing their focus on the everyday conduct of Danish citizens. From a remarkably stable mix of social welfarist and classical liberal rationalities, public health policies saw an infusion of what we call constructivist neoliberalism (Triantafillou, 2017, ch. 3). This does not amount to a wholesale abandonment of the former mix, but it does mean that both the social welfarist and the classical liberal rationalities are losing authority. The 1990s saw a number of changes whereby this mix no longer constitutes the sole nor even the most dominant form of political rationality in the area of public health. By the turn of the century, public health policies were increasingly informed by a constructivist neoliberalism that takes the capacities of communities, workplaces, families, and individuals to take care of their health by themselves as a precondition for handling health problems (Vallgårda, 2003).

Information campaigns and targeted taxes had for a long time played an important role in making Danes reduce their consumption of tobacco and alcohol. In the 1980s these instruments were supplemented with restrictions on children's access to these substances and regulations on their commercial advertisement (Vallgårda, 2003, p. 198). At the end of the decade, the Liberal–Conservative government launched a 'preventive programme' which argued that: 'It is the obligation of society to provide the basis for making the healthy choice easy; but even considerable efforts in the areas under the control of society cannot solve the health problems caused by the individual's lifestyle' (Sundhedsministeriet, 1989b, p. 11). The key challenge articulated by the programme was striking a balance between costly curative treatment and preventive treatment that risked 'wrap[ping] the population up in cotton' (Sundhedsministeriet, 1989b, p. 8). If preventive strategies, despite their anti-liberal connotations, were desirable or even necessary, it was because they held the promise of curbing the large and rising fiscal costs of public health policies (Sundhedsministeriet, 1989a, p. 20). Such costs were rising, it was argued, partly because of widespread diseases (cardiovascular and cancer) that in turn were attributable to the Danes' choice of lifestyle. Accordingly, even if the choice of lifestyle is an individual one and even if notions of a good life vary from one person to the next, society – a Danish euphemism for public authorities – should play a substantial role in providing the conditions for making the right choice of a healthy lifestyle (Sundhedsministeriet, 1989a, p. 11). Such interventions could include a wide range of sectors such as traffic, housing, environment, education, etc. that target those at risk (Sundhedsministeriet, 1989a, p. 9). The Liberal–Conservative coalition government then fundamentally recast the existing predominantly curative approach in favour of a potentially totalizing preventive approach targeting the sum of social environments shaping the choice of individual lifestyle.

The Healthy Cities Network, inaugurated in 1991, was probably the first comprehensive health promotion intervention in Denmark. Originally launched as an international network of municipalities inspired by the WHO's Health for All by the Year 2000 strategy and the subsequent Ottawa Charter described above, the national Healthy Cities Network was established with support from the Danish government under the banners of 'health promotion' and improving the 'quality of life'. The network emphasized 'health promotion and prevention of illness so as to support citizens in their full use of their physical, mental and social possibilities' (Dansk Institut for Klinisk Epidemiologi, 1998, p. 20) and argued that public health policies 'should not only prolong life but, to an equal measure, promote quality of life' (Dansk Institut for Klinisk Epidemiologi, 1998, p. 16). Another conceptual innovation derived from the WHO was that the linkage between health and the social and physical environment – the so-called *supportive environment* – should play an important role in health promotion work (Dansk Institut for Klinisk Epidemiologi, 1998, pp. 16–17). This environment was to ensure that the everyday life of each and every citizen was thoroughly embedded in codes of conduct and expert advice on how best to conduct oneself in a healthy way. In line with the WHO's Health for All by the Year 2000 strategy, municipalities that joined the Healthy City Network had to formulate and decide on preventive and health promotion policies and develop plans for making local citizens participate in debates on health issues (Dansk Institut for Klinisk Epidemiologi, 1998, pp. 108–112). The programme initially focused on the workplace but later spread to schools, communities, and families, with the key strategy of trying to 'anchor' processes of reflection leading to healthier styles of living in these various institutions (Frandsen and Triantafillou, 2011). At its peak in 2009, the network had grown to encompass 67 of 98 municipalities, and two out of five regions were members of the network. By early 2016, these numbers had dropped to 55 and one respectively (Sund By Netværket, 2016). The causes for this decline are not clear, but may very well have to do with the fact that many of the initiatives of the Network were taken over by the municipalities following the 2007 structural reform.

The shift in Danish public health towards health promotion during the 1990s was not only informed by the new WHO strategy. It was also underpinned by the emergence of systematic comparative epidemiological surveys illuminating the relatively poor health of the Danish population in comparison with improvements in public health in other European countries. In 1989, a report by the Danish Institute for Clinical Epidemiology (Dansk Institut for Klinisk Epidemiologi, DIKE) pointed to the 'surprisingly bad' development of average life expectancy and mortality in Denmark during the 1980s (Dansk Institut for Klinisk Epidemiologi, 1989).[3] A few years later the Average Life Expectancy Board was established under the Danish Ministry of Health in order to identify causes for the stagnating growth in average life expectancy of the Danish population (Dansk Institut for Klinisk Epidemiologi, 1993). In a dozen reports, the Board noted that the average life expectancy, health profile, and an average number of years of 'good' living of the Danish population were analysed and compared with the populations of other Western European countries. While the reports did not come up with any specific proposals for policy action, they left the clear impression that political action had to be taken to improve the life expectancy of the Danish population and that such actions could no longer rely on curative interventions only. The politicians had to devise a strategy that would target the everyday conduct or lifestyle of Danish citizens.

In 1999, the Social Democratic and Social Liberal government published a ten-year public health programme. The key problem identified was that the Danish population's health had failed to improve at the same rate as those of comparable industrialized nations (Sundhedsministeriet, 1999). Taking its cue from the WHO strategy Health for Everyone in the 21st Century, which insisted on promoting the health of everyone through their entire life, a wide range of tools seeking to improve health in people's everyday situations at school or workplace are suggested. In line with a number of comprehensive and comparative epidemiological surveys conducted in the early 1990s (Dansk Institut for Klinisk Epidemiologi, 1993), the programme paid particular attention to those diseases with the strongest impact on death rates and life expectancy, namely cardiovascular diseases, cancer, and sexually transmitted diseases (HIV/AIDS). As in Britain under the Blair government, socioeconomic inequality was regarded as a problem deserving specific attention, not because the poor do not have access to public health services, but because they are most likely to adopt an unhealthy lifestyle that puts them at particular risk: they smoke and drink more, exercise less, and their diet is not healthy. As physical coercion is out the question, the big challenge becomes: how to make the poor and less educated change their lifestyle by themselves? Notwithstanding the quest to make Danish citizens adopt a healthy lifestyle, it remained problematic throughout the 1990s for public authorities to intervene in individual conduct with reference to the risks linked to smoking and drinking. For example, it produced a public outcry when at the beginning of 2000 the Minister of Health suggested on national television that the new preventive health strategy in his opinion might very well entail that smoking ought to be banned in all public spaces. In fact, the Minister of Health resigned shortly after.

Yet the reluctance to interfere in the conduct of citizens with reference to the impact this could have on their health would change with surprising speed (Frandsen and Triantafillou, 2011). While the Danish preventive health strategies of the 1990s were still largely focused on risk behaviour and thereby implicitly seemed to be supported by a negative notion of health, the Healthy Throughout Life programme, launched in 2002 by the new Liberal–Conservative government, was informed by a positive notion of health. The key goal of the Liberal government's health programme, increasing average life expectancy, was identical to that of the Social Democratic government (Regeringen, 2002, p. 6). Apart from retaining the preventive approach targeting risk behaviour, the programme added that the quality of life must be improved at all its stages. In order to ensure the new political goals of health promotion, both the curative and the preventive strategies became inadequate.

Public authorities were now to deal not only with those already sick and those at risk but in principle with everyone during their entire life span.

Informed by this comprehensive health promotion ambition, the Liberal–Conservative government formed the Commission on Preventive Health Care in 2007 to prepare a new national Preventive Health Care programme with a view towards expanding average life expectancy and the quality of life of the Danish population (Forebyggelseskommissionen, 2009, pp. 6–8). In early 2009, the Commission published a lengthy report, *We Can Live Longer and Healthier*, containing a comprehensive set of recommendations including increased taxes on tobacco, alcohol, sweets, and animal fats, and VAT reductions on fruit and vegetables. It recommended smoke-free environments, warnings on tobacco products, age limits for sales of alcohol, prohibition of alcohol commercials, limited opening hours for tobacco sales, and food labelling assisting the consumer in the choice of healthy food. Moreover, physical planning and architecture should be designed to stimulate physical exercise. Individuals should be offered stop-smoking courses, treatment for alcoholism, and exercise prescriptions. Finally, the Commission endorsed 'arena-specific' interventions (such as fruit and healthy food in schools, teaching about healthy lifestyles, physical activities in schools and workplaces, after-school centres, and youth education institutions) and early 'tracking down' of risk behaviour through the municipal health services (Forebyggelseskommissionen, 2009). Many of the proposals met with intense public criticism for their illiberal implications, and so far very few have been adopted. Thus, classical liberal concerns over the individual's liberty from state intervention still play a significant role in Danish public health politics. Yet these suggestions do indicate just how far the thinking in Denmark about public health has moved within a decade or so, from one primarily orientated towards environmental and curative measures to one focusing on preventive measures, directly targeting individual conduct in the name of health promotion.

In sum, Danish public health policies underwent a significant mutation during the 1990s with the advent of health promotion strategies. The former reliance on a mix of curative strategies targeting the individual sufferer and preventive strategies targeting the physical environment was importantly supplemented and partially recast by rationalities seeking to promote the health of everyone. This strategic shift had at least two important implications. Firstly, in contrast to the relatively well-defined and numerically limited target group of the curative strategies, health promotion considerably expanded the target group to include anyone deemed at risk. As risk is a relative term – meaning that we are all at risk, though at significantly different levels; health promotion is really targeting every Dane, though in practice particular attention has been devoted to those considered as belonging to high-risk groups, such as smokers, the obese, alcohol abusers, the old, the poor, and those with very little education. Secondly, even if earlier preventive strategies targeting the physical environment aimed at improving the hygienic standards of each and every citizen, these interventions did not directly target the citizen. In contrast, health promotion directly targets the citizen's subjectivity and encourages her to work with herself in order to adopt different conduct. While health promotion is a liberal strategy that works through freedom, it is a much more direct form of power than earlier forms of prevention in that it directly engages with citizens' abilities to govern themselves.

Mobilizing communities in health promotion

This section examines how in both countries, though in different ways, the community was invoked in the attempt to promote the health of citizens.

England

The birth of health promotion in England has been closely linked to the attempt to mobilize the self-steering capacities of communities. Thus, health promotion is not only – or even primarily – about the individualization of the responsibility for choosing a healthy lifestyle but also about developing a community that renders the choice of a healthy lifestyle an easier one.

Britain has a long tradition of community health projects, mostly targeting poor neighbourhoods, going back to the 1930s, with the most famous example being the Peckham experiment in southeast London (Pearse and Crocker, 2007 [1943]). While this private initiative was followed by other attempts to provide health services and stimulate local citizens to engage in physical exercise and healthy eating, they seemed not to be part of a public health strategy. It is not until the establishment of Community Health Councils in 1974 that we see the emergence of a state-orchestrated strategy of invoking the community in matters of health politics (Baggott, 2013, pp. 99–100). In cooperation with the NHS, Community Health Councils were to monitor local health conditions, provide information on available local health services, suggest improvements, and assist with complaints. However, during the 1980s and 1990s, the Councils were increasingly ignored by the NHS. This was not to signal the end of the ideal of community participation in health promotion. With the advent of the New Labour government a bewildering set of local agencies and networks were established, including Patient Advice and Liaison Services, Independent Complaints

Advocacy Services, and Patient and Public Involvement Forums. Their combined role was to coordinate local interventions and mobilize local resources to provide more equal access to health services and promote healthy conduct. Not surprisingly, their efforts were criticized for being fragmented and not very effective in improving health in vulnerable communities (Hogg, 2009).

A wide number of concrete interventions seeking to make citizens reduce alcohol consumption, adopt a better diet, and engage in physical exercise were conducted via government programmes. In the following we account for the key strategies and techniques of government employed in three of these programmes, namely: Sure Start, Healthy Living Centres, and Communities for Health. The Sure Start programmes were launched around 1997/98 as a national initiative targeting preschool children and their families in disadvantaged areas (Gidley, 2007). The Sure Start programmes financed several interventions, but health improvement was one of the major components. Moreover, the emphasis was on preventive rather than curative strategies in order to make families better equipped to attend to the health of their children and make them adopt a healthy lifestyle. By providing equal access to health advice, training, and services to all families in a given (deprived) area, Sure Start deliberately tried to avoid the potentially stigmatizing effects of needs-based interventions (Gidley, 2007, p. 148). On the one hand, then, the Sure Start programme retained the kind of liberal rationales that seek to invoke the responsibility of parents in order to improve the health of children. On the other hand, it partially broke with such classical liberal rationales and instead operated with communitarian logic that regarded the community and its empowering capacities as the key agent of health promotion. Thus, rather than trying to implement uniform programmes, communities – through the assistance of Children's Centres – were urged to build partnerships among local actors and design the interventions according to what they saw as the most urgent local health needs (Gidley, 2007, p. 149).

The Healthy Living Centre programme was set up in 1998 to fund community-level interventions to address health inequalities and improve health and wellbeing (Hills et al., 2007). The programme funded 351 Healthy Living Centres all over Britain, which in turn generated a wide range of different activities targeting local communities. A part of these activities operated within one central building, while others served as hubs for partnerships or networks of activities run by different organizations at a number of different sites. Some Centres focused on providing specific health-related services; however, many addressed wider issues, such as social isolation, unemployment, and poverty, as these were seen to influence the health of local citizens. Again, it is possible to distinguish between activities targeting individuals and their lifestyle, on the one hand, and interventions targeting the community and its capacity to assist and mobilize the health of its citizens on the other. Individualizing measures included advice on diet, smoking cessation, and alcohol abuse, practical training in cooking and physical exercise, and various therapeutic interventions seeking to increase the self-esteem of citizens (Hills et al., 2007, pp. 51–56). Initiatives targeting the community and its capacity included the provision of services that were easily accessible to local groups, in the language of the community, and intensive and personalized (Hills et al., 2007, pp. 75–80). Moreover, it entailed home visits or outreach into groups already working with the community. Finally, in order to create sustainable capacity-building, community action teams and lay health workers (educators) were trained to continue the task of assisting other local citizens in improving their health.

The making of community health educators is particularly interesting, as the making of these educators is exemplary for the rationality informing the exercise of power in health promotion. Community health educator programmes date back to at least the early 1990s and became regarded by Blair's New Labour government as crucial for building sustainable community capacity in health promotion (Chiu, 2003). Today, Community Educator programmes are found across the UK, though their number remains unknown (South, White, and Gamsu, 2013, p. 102). In order to become a health educator it is necessary to go through a 14-week course that focuses not only on medical knowledge but also – much more importantly – on the personal development of the health educator (South et al., 2013, p. 108). In order to enable educators to act as connectors between local citizens and relevant health services and, more generally, as facilitators of local resources and citizen empowerment, the training emphasizes that they are not to become medical experts but coaches or empowerment agents. This model, inspired by Brazilian educator Paolo Freire, implies that the gaze and the governing activity of the educator must be targeted not only at other local citizens but also herself. The educator must be willing and able to build up her own confidence and constantly reflect on her own role vis-à-vis other local citizens. It is only by giving up the role of the all-knowing expert and adopting the reflexive role of the facilitator, it is argued, that she can really engage with local citizens and make sure that power is transferred to the disempowered. In brief, the empowerment of the community hinges on the making of educators or facilitators willing to make themselves the object of intervention by themselves. It is this ethos and practical reflexive work of self-government that forms the foundation for the educator's ability to empower others and, ultimately, the entire community. A slightly different manifestation of this programme was continued by the Coalition government under the heading of Community Health Champions (NHS Confederation and AllTogetherBetter, 2012).

The Communities for Health programme was launched in 2004 in order to enhance the capacity of communities to make individuals adopt a healthier lifestyle, build partnerships between health organizations and communities, and develop innovative practices reducing health inequality (Baggott, 2013, p. 114). Some 360 activities and interventions were implemented in 80 local authority areas and targeted smoking, alcohol, obesity, and sexual health. The focus was explicitly aimed at enhancing health and wellbeing rather than curing particular diseases, a strategy that was deemed successful by external evaluations (Local Government Association, 2011). Finally, in order to reinvigorate the attempt to engage the community in health promotion, Patient and Public Involvement Forums were replaced in 2008 by the so-called LINks, a social care and health service providing institution run by local governments (Baggott, 2013, pp. 101–102). However, it seems that LINks did not fare much better than its predecessors in mobilizing local communities or equalizing health conditions. At any rate, the advent of the Coalition government meant that LINks was replaced in 2012 by Health Watch England and its local affiliates, which were given the task of providing health advice to individual citizens, information about available health services, and advice on how to complain in case the latter services were deemed insufficient (Baggott, 2013, pp. 106–107).

Apart from emphasizing the role of local authorities, the Coalition government envisaged that workplace employers and local food markets were to play an important role in contributing to healthier environments and – for the latter – in offering wholesome foods for local citizens. In line with the Blair government's partnership strategy, the Coalition government established Health and Wellbeing Boards charged with providing oversight of the local health and care system. This included producing: joint strategic needs assessments of the current and future health and social care needs of the local population; joint health and wellbeing strategies for meeting the local health needs identified in the needs assessments; and overseeing the so-called Better Care Fund plans seeking to better integrate local health and social care services.

Many community health promotion programmes launched under New Labour were terminated either by default or by design with the advent of the Coalition government. However, the communitarian rationale by which communities were designated as sites of intervention and health empowering activities remained important. Thus the establishment of Public Health England explicitly aimed at enhancing the role of local governments in promoting community-based health initiatives (e.g. Local Government Association and Public Health England, 2014).

In sum, there has been a consistent concern in England for the mobilization of the community in the quest for promoting the health of the English populace. Of course, we should be very careful not to exaggerate the rigour and scale of the programmes constituting this quest. As repeated in several evaluation reports, most of these programmes merely undertake information campaigns and one-way consultations. Yet the ambition of politicians, health professionals, and academics in the field is clearly more ambitious than that. Moreover, their limitations notwithstanding, many programmes are both comprehensive in their scope and target the conduct of individuals in a very direct way. Above all, for all the institutional turmoil and fragmentation following the shift of governments, there is a constant concern over how to make programmes reach communities more effectively and augment their capacity to promote health and make local citizens adopt healthier lifestyles.

Denmark

In 2007, the Danish political-administrative system underwent its largest transformation since 1970. The so-called structural reform entailed a massive centralization of all the major welfare services. Thus, the number of counties – with the key task of running public hospitals and regulating the conditions of private general practitioners – was reduced from 14 to only 5 so-called regions. The number of municipalities was reduced from 275 to 98, and by the same token the municipalities were charged with a new responsibility, namely to undertake preventive and health promotion interventions.

From the very outset of the structural reform, municipalities have complained almost incessantly both over inadequate resources and guidelines on how to effectively engage in health promotion. In order to help the municipalities in their new task, the Danish Health Authority (Sundhedsstyrelsen) issued a dozen 'prevention packages' in 2012 covering areas such as physical exercise, tobacco habits, obesity, diet, mental health, sexual health, sun protection, etc. (Sundhedsstyrelsen, 2012a, 2012b, 2012c, 2012d, 2013). Each package explains in some detail the prevalence of the health issue to be dealt with by the municipality, the direct and indirect costs of the health problem, the legal regulations in the area, the medical evidence of the efficacy of existing interventions, municipal experiences, and the Danish Health Authority's recommended guidelines for intervention in the area. Most importantly, the packages all point to the need for cooperation and partnerships between the municipality and local public and private organizations, such as schools, other educational institutions, sports clubs, gymnastic associations, and workplaces. To encourage and individualize municipalities' preventive and health promotion efforts, they were given access to individualized information about the health of their citizens based on the national health profile, a database formed around the unique Danish centralized person register (Rigsrevisionen, 2013). A survey of the preventive and health promotion efforts undertaken by 11 Danish municipalities in the period 2007–2011 showed that all had a strong focus on better diet, boosting physical exercise, and reducing alcohol and tobacco consumption (Rigsrevisionen, 2013). It also documented the impact that the structural reform had on municipalities' efforts in these areas. Some municipalities had begun activities in this area prior to the 2007 reform, and all had significantly stepped up their initiatives following the reform. However, the survey also showed not only that the level of engagement varied significantly between the municipalities but also that the Ministry of Health's monitoring of the municipal actions in this area was not very thorough.

In early 2014, the Social Democrat-led coalition government issued seven goals for the population's health standards over the ensuing ten years (Regeringen, 2014). The overall goal was raising the number of quality life years for the entire Danish population. The seven concrete goals were to: reduce the inequality within the population's health status; improve the mental health of children; improve the mental health of adults; reduce tobacco consumption; reduce alcohol damage and youth alcohol use; reduce child obesity; and increase everyday physical exercise. These goals largely echo those propagated since the 1990s. Moreover, in line with the prevention packages from 2012, the national plan formulated a 'partnership strategy' emphasizing the cooperation between a wide range of public and private actors. Apart from hospitals, municipalities, and the individual citizen, the 'partnership strategy' was to mobilize schools, sports clubs, workplaces, trade unions, employers, insurance companies, universities, and other organizations. They were to join forces in order to come up with new ideas, develop shared attitudes towards health, implement local initiatives, and share their experiences (Regeringen, 2014, pp. 22–23). In sum, the only way to increase the population's average number of healthy life years is through a concerted effort of public and private actors in which everyone has a responsibility to promote the population's health. While the plan does emphasize the individual's responsibility to take care of her life and choose a healthy lifestyle, it does not mention the possible political problems implied by a strategy seeking to make everyone change their lifestyle.

If the move towards health promotion has been mainly driven by public authorities, notably the Ministry of Health, the Health Authority, and, a bit later on, the municipalities, private organizations have also played an important role. Here it is important to note that Denmark has a very large voluntary sector, with huge membership. In the context of health promotion, one organization is particularly important: the Danish Gymnastics and Sports Association (Danske Gymnastik- og Idrætsforeninger, DGI). The DGI was established in 1861 with a view towards encouraging popular gymnastics and mobilizing rifle shooters in the mounting war against Prussia over the duchies of Holstein, Lauenburg, and Schleswig. In the decades following the lost war, the rifle-shooting faction would gradually lose importance vis-à-vis the increasingly popular gymnastics movement. While physical exercise, together with cultural formation, played a key rationale of the DGI throughout the twentieth century, it was never directly integrated into biopolitical interventions, i.e. the efforts of the Danish state to secure its population's health and vigour. It was only at the end of the 2000s that DGI decided to link with the state's health promotion strategy. Following drops in membership rates and government plans to put the municipalities in charge of preventive strategies and health promotion (DGI, 2005), the DGI decided not only to include the promotion of public health as one of its key organizational targets (Vucina, 2014, p. 173). It also embarked on several initiatives to cooperate with municipalities on efforts to make Danes more physically active (DGI, 2011, pp. 27, 33–35). At the local level, a number of sports clubs, voluntary organizations, and private workplaces have in various ways been engaged in projects with the municipal health services in various health promotion initiatives.

In brief, health promotion around the mid-2010s in Denmark broadly revolves around a two-pronged strategy: one series of interventions targeting specific individuals with health problems or deemed at risk and another series targeting the environment of each and every Dane with a view towards making them adopt a healthier lifestyle. It is this second prong that is fundamentally new and perhaps also the most politically problematic element of the current health promotion strategy. To intervene in the environment is not only or even primarily about changing the physical surroundings, such as the creation of bike lanes, playgrounds, exercise trails, etc., but more about creating a dense network of collaborating organizations propagating codes of conduct and practical knowledge about how to live a healthy life.

Conclusion

In this chapter we have tried to account for key events constituting the development of modern biopower in England and Denmark. The focus has been on the strategies employed to improve the health of citizens and the rationalities informing these. We have also briefly touched on key organizational designs in the unfolding of public health strategies. We found remarkable similarities between the two countries but also some important differences.

In both England and Denmark, the emergence of modern biopower, whereby the state assumes responsibility for the health and wellbeing of its population, took place during the nineteenth century. Both countries are unitary states, and both offer extensive public health services that are largely funded by taxation. We found that two strategies played a particularly important role in both countries throughout the nineteenth and most of the twentieth century: preventive strategies via modifications of the physical environment to promote hygiene and curative strategies seeking to make public health services available to all citizens. Negative eugenics constituted a distinct preventive strategy in both countries during the first half of the twentieth century. However, the strategy of preventing the procreation of the feeble-minded played out quite differently in the two countries. In England, negative eugenics remained at the level of scientific discourse and political debate; in Denmark, it resulted in the legal sanctioning of sterilization, abortions, and restriction of marriage.

Both countries saw the emergence of health promotion during the 1990s. This new strategy was gradually developed from around 1990 in response partly to WHO's Ottawa Charter and partly to national epidemiological studies that visualized stalling life expectancy and rapid increases in the incidence of cardiovascular, oncological, and endocrinological diseases. Under the banner of stimulating lifestyle changes, this new biopolitical strategy is above all characterized by working through the self-steering capacities of individuals and of communities (or more broadly, the environment). A number of interventions have been launched in both countries to enhance the capacity of those individuals and communities deemed at risk to govern themselves more effectively in accordance with contemporary norms of health. Three points are worth stressing here. Firstly, contemporary health promotion differs importantly from both curative and earlier preventive approaches precisely because it works through the active participation and, thereby, the subjectivity of individuals and communities. Secondly, health promotion is not only or even primarily about charging individuals with the responsibility for their own health with a view towards legitimizing the withdrawal of public health services, though this does seem to have played a role – in particular in England after 2010. Rather, health promotion is about targeting both individuals and the wider institutional environment (often termed community) to create a grid in which healthy lifestyle choice becomes easier and, conversely, making the choice of supposedly wrong lifestyles more difficult. Thirdly, resistance against health promotion in both countries has tended to focus rather narrowly either on the ban on alcohol and tobacco sales and consumption or on the stigmatization of (mostly poor) people with an unhealthy lifestyle. Very few have criticized the attempt to governmentalize the life of individuals and their institutional environments (family, peers, workplace, school, sports club, supermarket, local government, etc.) in order to improve the lifestyle of all.

With regard to community empowerment, or the governmentalization of the institutional environment of citizens, it may be noted that both countries have a strong tradition of non-profit, private organizations contributing to the provision of various social activities and services. However, classical liberal rationalities seem to play a stronger role in England than in Denmark, in the sense of a strong political and public preference for private (both profit and non-profit) organizations involved in health service provision. In Denmark, local neighbourhoods and voluntary organizations have played a very important role too, but in most concrete programmes their mandates and activities are shaped by municipalities, which are charged with formal responsibility for health promotion. This may have to do with a relatively strong Danish corporatist tradition, in which institutionalized dialogue between public and select private actors is envisaged to be conducive to effective policymaking (P. Christiansen and Nørgaard, 2002). The similarities and the differences between the English and Danish forms of health promotion will become clearer in the following chapters, in which we examine the control of obesity and the recovery approach to mental illness.

Notes

1 This section draws on Triantafillou (2012, pp. 98–100).
2 According to the BIT homepage, organ donation seems to constitute the only systematic attempt to employ nudging in the area of health promotion (Behavioural Insights Team, 2016).
3 The Danish Institute for Clinical Epidemiology changed its name to the State Institute for Public Health (Statens Institut for Folkesundhed) in 1999. The latter is located at the University of Southern Denmark, Odense.

3
Fighting obesity in England

As in many other OECD countries, obesity has been a major concern of public authorities in England since the 1990s. In October 2007, the Secretary of State for Health, Alan Johnson, stated that obesity constituted a 'potential crisis on the scale of climate change' (BBC News, 2007). Four years before that the Chief Medical Officer for England, Sir Liam Donaldson, had issued the following dramatic declaration:

> The growth of overweight and obesity in the population of our country – particularly amongst children – is a major concern. It is a health time bomb with the potential to explode over the next three decades ... Unless this time bomb is defused the consequences for the population's health, the costs to the NHS and losses to the economy will be disastrous. (Department of Health, 2003, p. 44)

Donaldson found it necessary to address this national problem with a wide range of initiatives ranging from more intense local monitoring of the prevalence of obesity, regulation of food products and labelling, training of health professionals in providing advice on obesity control, the singling out of children showing early signs of obesity, and local government action programmes (Department of Health, 2003, p. 44). Many of these recommendations were taken up by the New Labour government and to some extent by the subsequent Coalition government.

A number of critical studies have been carried out on the politics of obesity emerging first in the US and later in many Western European countries. Some of these focus on the exaggerated claims about the negative effects of obesity (e.g. Campos, 2004; J. Oliver, 2006). These studies argue that scientists and pharmaceutical companies have conspired to exaggerate if not the prevalence then the negative health effects of obesity in order to boost the demand for their medical products. We do not engage with this argument as our concern here is with problematizing the kind of power exercised over or through citizens, not whether this power is legitimate (as in medically justified).

Others have pointed to the powerful effect of the quantified construct Body Mass Index (BMI) and its complicity in lending legitimacy to interventions in the lives of people objectified as obese (B. Evans and Colls, 2009). Along the same lines, others have pointed to the negative and stigmatizing effects that obesity discourses have on the lives of people defined as obese (Gard and Wright, 2005). Some have pointed out the many ways in which young people resist current medical ideals about the body and its weight (Coffey, Budgeon, and Cahill, 2016). Yet again, such studies tend to regard the obese (and the underweight) as the objects of a reductionist medical gaze underpinned by an oppressive apparatus of medical power.

While we agree that the label of obesity may in some cases be stigmatizing, we will show in this chapter that the medical power pursued in contemporary obesity policies is not only or even primarily objectifying and repressive. On the contrary, most policies are voluntary and work through self-subjectification. True, the medical discourses around obesity are no doubt objectifying the obese; however, the ensuing interventions are not trying to impose a disciplinary scheme on a passive target group but rather to stimulate the latter to reflect on their choice of lifestyle and how to change it. In fact, several studies have criticized the overwhelming focus in obesity policies on individual responsibility at the expense of economic and social factors (e.g. Cain, 2013). Finally, a few studies have pointed to the expanding and seemingly limitless character of contemporary obesity discourses in the sense that they identify and target in the present those who are calculated as potential patients in the future (B. Evans and Colls, 2011). That is, all citizens are regarded at – various levels of – risk of becoming obese, which makes us all potential targets of obesity control interventions. We agree that this is certainly a danger of the new lifestyle approach, and this danger is motivating the analysis in this chapter of the political rationalities and some of the many programmes and techniques employed in the fight against obesity.

Our main argument in this chapter is that the so-called neoliberal health policies pursued since the 1990s have entailed the making of a comprehensive apparatus of central and local authorities teaming up with voluntary organizations and for-profit organizations to govern in the name of the community. Thus, obesity control in England does not merely imply that the responsibility for obesity is individualized in the sense of simply being delegated to citizens themselves. It also, at least ideally, implies the establishment of a far-reaching apparatus that seeks to shape the institutional environment that in turn impinges on the everyday choice of lifestyle. This apparatus has largely failed when judged by its own terms, i.e. the reduction of obesity in England. Yet it has succeeded in the sense that the persistence of obesity has resulted in calls for more interventions to empower communities and their citizens rather than less.

At the most general level, this chapter analyses predominant forms of political rationalities, expert knowledge, and governing technologies employed in the attempt to govern obesity in England.

More specifically, we look in the first section at some of the historical antecedents to contemporary health promotion by briefly accounting for the preventive measures addressing obesity in the early twentieth century. We then turn to the invention or, rather, recasting of obesity as a question of lifestyle conduct during the 1980s. This is followed by an examination of the mobilization of the community by the Blair government's fight against obesity. We then turn to the Cameron government's reinvention of the role of communities and the attempt to apply behavioural knowledge and techniques to governing obesity. Finally, we zoom in on a specific site of intervention, namely the governing of child obesity and the role that so-called fat camps play in obesity management.

Historical antecedents

Judging from the many government reports and also from some of the academic studies of the politics of obesity, it may seem that obesity only became a concern for government from the 1990s. Yet the fight against obesity in England has a longer history. Our aim here is not to unravel the genealogy of obesity in Britain, but firstly to specify the uniqueness of current English obesity control and, secondly to make the point that the political concern over obesity cannot simply be explained in terms of biomedical concerns over the growth of the prevalence of obesity. Rather, the political concern with obesity is linked with wider governmental rationalities and biopolitical concerns over the vigour and quality of the English population and, ultimately, the productivity and competitiveness of the British labour force and economy.

In its modern form, the political concern over obesity dates back to the 1870s, when various representatives of the medical profession would problematize not only the thin and undernourished, but also, more surprisingly, overweight citizens (Zweiniger-Bargielowska, 2005). Over the next 60 years, England would see a growing interest in diet, physical practices, and self-discipline through medical writings, a rising market of popular self-help guides, press coverage of fitness and physical culture, and, ultimately, a government-driven health and fitness campaign in the late 1930s. This attention to obesity and to a lesser extent constipation was linked to growing eugenic concerns over the quality of the British race, which was seen as endangered by the rising number of obese and physically degenerate middle-class urban citizens with primarily sedentary work. The Chief Medical Officer to the Ministry of Health, George Newman, would argue in 1929 that building a healthy race was one of the key objects of government (Ministry of Health, 1929, pp. 206–208). This was followed in the late 1930s by a comprehensive government campaign for physical exercise and better diet and the Physical Training and Recreation Act of 1937, which granted money to local authorities and voluntary organizations for the construction of physical recreation facilities (Zweiniger-Bargielowska, 2005, pp. 250–251). While the development of a British physical culture movement during the early twentieth century and the national fitness campaign of the late 1930s may have epistemic affinities with eugenic notions of race improvement, they explicitly rejected authoritarian rule and negative strategies, such as obstructing procreation. Much as in Denmark, the emphasis was on positive eugenics, i.e. the constant vigilance over and development of the body's physical abilities by way of health education and social reforms. The ambition was not to develop a superior race but to improve the health of workers and soldiers and, thereby, to contribute to national efficiency and strength (Jones, 1986; Zweiniger-Bargielowska, 2006).

We want to stress two points here. Firstly, the government interventions employed generally worked within a liberal register in the sense that their key strategies were to rely on citizens freely adopting healthier forms of conduct through a combination of information campaigns and the provision of physical exercise facilities. The most direct form of intervention took place in schools and the Boy Scout movement, where initiatives were taken to boost physical training and a sense of the importance of proper diet. Secondly, it is telling that this early concern over obesity peaked during the 1930s in the midst of a period of mass unemployment and poverty in British society where many had problems providing daily meals. In demographic and epidemiological terms obesity was really a minor health issue and therefore the political concern over obesity could not be reduced to a narrow biomedical concern or to some pre-discursive reality of obesity. This early concern with obesity only makes sense if we take into account wider biopolitical concerns over the quality of the British stock or population and its immanent fear of degeneration nurtured by eugenic discourses at the time.

Recasting obesity as an issue of lifestyle regulation

Obesity took a long time to re-emerge on the political agenda in England. While a few spectacular attempts were made to problematize the link between nutrition and health during the 1980s, it would take another decade before obesity was taken up as an object of systematic government intervention. This time, though, it was addressed not in terms of stock and heredity but in terms of lifestyle.

In 1983, a provocative report on the status of nutrition was made public after attempts by the Conservative government to withhold it (C. Walker and Cannon, 1985). The report was prepared for the National Advisory Committee on Nutrition Education (NACNE), which had been established by Margaret Thatcher in 1979 in order to provide simple and accurate information on nutrition. An expert group, a sub-committee of NACNE, was set up in 1980 to review the findings of recent official reports and publications and to make recommendations. The NACNE report addressed obesity as well as cardiovascular disease and indicated that other diseases were also preventable by a healthy diet. In line with the recent ideas about 'the whole-population' approach formulated by the WHO, it argued that confining attention to 'at-risk groups' was an error.[1] It formulated quantified targets for reduction in the intake of fats, sugars, and salt and increases in starchy foods, vegetables, and fruits. Moreover, the report proposed legislation and regulation to encourage breeding of lean animals, require explicit nutritional labelling, and reformulate fatty processed foods. The report received a lot of media attention because it linked, in a rather frank manner, the average British diet and heightened risks of developing colorectal cancer, diabetes, hypertension, and stroke. The report was followed by the development of official guidelines for healthy eating, and attempts were made to educate adults and schoolchildren in accordance with these guidelines by way of general information campaigns. However, no systematic attempts were made to intervene more directly in the eating and physical behaviour of citizens.

The Conservative government in England would later acknowledge that obesity was a threat to the health of the nation – by its complicity with the high prevalence of coronary diseases – that called for specific action. While this strategy was ground-breaking in making health promotion a key aim of public health policies and while it did propose new actions, the scope of the latter remained quite limited, and the results of these were disappointing. Thus, the target set in the Health of the Nation strategy to reduce the prevalence of obesity among adults to 7 per cent (based on 1986/87 levels) by 2005 (Secretary of State for Health, 1992, p. 20) was not reached. True, a concerted strategy involving central and local government and public and private actors was launched to make the English adopt a healthier diet and engage in more physical exercise. As mentioned in Chapter 2, these interventions depended entirely on voluntary mechanisms, such as information, guidelines, and care services. More direct forms of interventions, such as bans on alcohol, duties on unhealthy food items, or changes in the urban environment to make people start walking or cycling, were either non-existent or very modest (Jebb, Aveyard, and Hawkes, 2013, p. 42).

The feeble efforts made by the Conservative government from the late 1980s notwithstanding, these efforts would define a strategy that would largely remain unaltered for the next three decades. In essence it rested on mobilizing the self-governing potential of individuals and the environments surrounding them. Conversely, except in very rare cases, this strategy avoided the use of coercive instruments such as bans or forced removal of children. Moreover, and more surprisingly, the fight against obesity would make very limited use of bariatric surgery in spite of mounting evidence of the comparative efficacy of surgery as against the various medical and behavioural interventions (Gloy et al., 2013). In fact, between 2011 and 2014, the number of surgeries fell from 8,794 to 6,032 (P. Brown, 2016). It has been estimated that the procedure is provided for much less than 1 per cent of obese people who could benefit in the UK (Gloy et al., 2013). Not surprisingly, the direct costs of surgery have been given as an explicit reason for limiting its use (Rawlinson and Johnston, 2016). However, concerns over costs and cost-effectiveness are hardly the main reason for insisting on the pursuit of preventive and health promotion strategies in as much as such calculations have rarely been made. Rather, as we will try to show in the following, the political insistence on prevention and promotion seems to have to do with a wider political rationality that holds a very strong faith in the effectiveness and moral desirability of making citizens and communities able to govern themselves properly, i.e. in accordance with contemporary ideals of health and weight.

Governing obesity through the environment

From the late 1990s, obesity and the diseases it causes started receiving increasing political attention. One of the reasons for this was the many epidemiological and biomedical studies published by the National Institute for Health Care and Excellence (NICE). These studies illuminated the growing prevalence of obesity in the British population and made visible many of its unfortunate medical effects on individual life and vigour (for an overview of NICE reports during the 2000s cf. Jebb et al., 2013).

Whatever the reason, obesity control rapidly became an important issue of the New Labour government. In 1999, it published the strategy document *Saving Lives: Our Healthier Nation*, which placed obesity control as a crucial object among the wider attempts to promote healthier lives (Secretary of State for Health, 1999). The report found obesity to be a serious problem and noted that in 1996, 61 per cent of men and 52 per cent of women were either overweight or obese. As part of its general health promotion strategy, New Labour argued in favour of 'integrated action' that would address people at all ages and, more importantly, the various social, economic, and environmental conditions that impinge on individual behaviour (Secretary of State for Health, 1999a, p. 53). This included employment, poverty, access to retailers of healthy food, and building social capital and cohesive communities. Apart from systematic dissemination of authoritative advice on proper diet and physical activity, the strategy promised to enhance cookery education at schools (Secretary of State for Health, 1999a, p. 37), expand affordable sports and leisure opportunities at local neighbourhood level (Secretary of State for Health, 1999a, p. 115), and enhance advice for first-time parents on child nutrition (Secretary of State for Health, 1999a, p. 116). Many of the local efforts were to be developed and coordinated by the establishment of Healthy Living Centres (see Chapter 2).

By 2001 the National Audit Office reported that obesity had trebled in England in the previous 20 years. It was highly critical of NHS strategies and programmes, which it described as 'patchy' (National Audit Office, 2001, p. 2). It thus found that while effective joined-up strategies had been adopted locally in a number of places in Britain, in most areas this was not the case. The National Audit Office formulated a number of recommendations to the government. For example, the Department of Health should reinforce the coordination of surveys and research by establishing a cross-departmental advisory group to coordinate all research on obesity and measures to prevent it (National Audit Office, 2001, p. 20). Moreover, the Department of Health should lead the development of an inter-departmental strategy to promote the health benefits of physical activity. Thirdly, together with the Department of the Environment, Transport, and the Regions, the Department of Health should encourage local authorities and health authorities to adopt local targets for cycling and walking to provide clear incentives to support healthy modes of travel. Fourthly, the efforts undertaken at state schools to make pupils engage in physical activity and learn about healthy nutrition and how to cook healthy food should be further expanded. In sum, the National Audit Office recommended a broad strategy including interventions in a wide range of settings in order to have an impact on the daily lives of the British people.

This comprehensive strategy was rearticulated in an even more systematic manner by way of the Foresight analysis issued by the Government Office for Science (Butland et al., 2007). Based on a complex systems approach, the Government Office for Science outlined an analytical model seeking to grasp the complex dynamics leading to obesity. The key explanatory variable emerging from this analytical model is the 'obesogenic environment' (Butland et al., 2007, p. 52). The latter term was invented a few years before by medical researchers trying to design preventive health care strategies targeting, among other things, obesity (Eggar and Swinburn, 2002). It is this environment, which in itself is the product of a complex set of factors, that causes individuals to take in more calories than they use. The Foresight analysis produced a complex series of diagrams for different population groups. The diagrams identify variables joined by 'causal' loops divided into seven interlinked areas: physiology, individual physical activity, physical activity environment, individual psychology, social psychology, food production, and food consumption. The 'causal loops' link these variables to a central 'obesity engine' that functions through a biological 'core balancing loop' that regulates body weight and a 'reinforcing loop' that overrides the core balancing loop when the social, physical, or technological environment 'short-circuits' the 'evolutionary driver … driving an incessant process of accumulation and conservation' (Butland et al., 2007, 2007, p. 80). These complex variables amount to produce more or less strong 'obesogenic environments' which, if not tackled by government interventions, will result in 60 per cent of the British population being overweight by 2050 (Butland et al., 2007, p. 23).

The Foresight analysis is interesting because it clearly does not reduce the problem of obesity to a question of individual lifestyle and thereby an individual moral responsibility. On the contrary, its analysis clears a space for government intervention that addresses a wide set of individual and, not least, social environments, such as the community. Thus, our point here is not that the Foresight analysis and its notion of obesogenic environment may amount to a form of 'environmental determinism', as argued by one critical scholar (B. Evans, 2010). Rather the point is that this kind of complex analysis invites a series of government interventions that go way beyond classical liberal interventions with their combined focus on curative strategies, such as the treatment provided by GPs and hospitals, and individual responsibility.

It has recently been argued that the very complexity of the factors involved in the Foresight study has somewhat paradoxically weakened attempts to regulate environmental and societal factors (Ulijaszek and McLennan, 2016, p. 407). While we agree that the focus on individual choice of (healthy or unhealthy) lifestyle has been a cornerstone of New Labour's health policy and probably even more so the policy of the Coalition government and the current Conservative government, this is hardly due to the Foresight analysis. Firstly, the Foresight analysis recommended five strands of intervention, of which only one is curative and the others are preventive: provide effective treatment and support when people become overweight or obese; promote children's health; promote healthy food; build physical activity into our lives; and support health at work and provide incentives more widely to promote health. In brief, the Foresight analysis encourages a set of interventions addressing both individual and social spheres, public and private settings – with the only political limitation being the technical capacity of existing government techniques to actually address these complex dynamics of obesity. It seems then that (classical) liberal qualms about the danger of excessive state intervention are far away from the horizon of public health policy.

Secondly, the Foresight analysis explicitly informed, but did not determine, New Labour's ensuing policy on obesity control. In January 2008, the government released its report *Healthy Weight, Healthy Lives*, which largely followed the lines of intervention suggested by the Foresight analysis. This entailed making children adopt a healthy lifestyle, promoting healthy food choice, building physical activity into the everyday life of citizens, creating incentives for workplaces to provide healthy settings for their employees, and providing individualized advice and service (Department of Health, 2008, pp. xii–xiv). Gordon Brown, the newly elected Prime Minister, explained that this strategy, on the one hand, emphasized choice and the responsibility of the individual for choosing a healthy lifestyle and, on the other hand, required government intervention to assist such choices by providing information, access to healthy food and exercise, and various health and social services (Department of Health, 2008, p. iii).

The *Healthy Weight, Healthy Lives* strategy proposed a number of mostly indirect and voluntary governing mechanisms to be employed at the five sites mentioned above. Firstly, the strategy targets children and young people in order to make durable lifestyle changes. Here the school is envisaged to play a key role by providing mandatory physical exercise and cookery lessons. For example, mandated nutritional standards for food were introduced in state-run schools in 2007. There is also a school fruit and vegetable scheme, in place since 2004, which provides fruits or vegetables each school day to children aged 4–6 years and compulsory cookery lessons for all 11- to 14-year-olds (Jebb et al., 2013, p. 52). Another major effort is the singling out of the very young child deemed at risk by addressing obese pregnant mothers and providing them with information on the importance of breastfeeding and proper diet for them and their children (Department of Health, 2008, pp. 7–17). First-time parents under the age of 20 years are also supported via the Family Nurse Partnership, a structured programme of home visits that includes support for breastfeeding and healthy weaning practices (Jebb et al., 2013).

Thirdly, in order to promote healthier food choices, the government would further develop its dialogue with the food industry to endorse healthy diet information and schemes, alter its labelling and marketing strategies, reduce the size of unhealthy food servings, and reduce the amount of sugar, fats, and salt in food commodities (Jebb et al., 2013, pp. 18–19). Further, with a view towards building in physical activity in everyday life of citizens, the government plans not only to launch campaigns for exercise but also to encourage national and local city planners to facilitate walking and cycling instead of driving (Jebb et al., 2013, pp. 19–22). Fourthly, attempts were made to enhance employers' incentives to provide healthy lifestyle choices for their employees, though this so far seems to be limited to the development of experimental pilot programmes with companies and engaging in dialogue with existing fitness centres on how to attract more active members. Finally, in order to improve the individualized service for citizens, the NHS and general practitioners were to offer obese people and other citizens deemed at risk both standard information packages and an individually tailored service (Jebb et al., 2013, pp. 24–26).

In brief, individualized interventions, such as information campaigns, expert counselling, health education, and various training programmes, seek to make each and every citizen take responsibility for conducting herself and her lifestyle in a healthy manner. Simultaneously, New Labour embarked on a strategy invoking the environment in general and the community in particular. This strategy aimed to create an institutional framework envisaged to empower communities and their citizens to take better care of themselves and their health. This strategy differed both from the traditional curative approach, whereby medical services were made available to sick citizens in need of a cure, and from the individualizing strategy, focusing only on empowering individuals and making them responsible for their health.

Behaviourist aspirations and reinvigoration of the community

As mentioned in the preceding chapter, the British public health services were subject to substantial budget cuts following the advent of the Cameron-led Coalition government in 2010. These cuts also affected the preventive services, including funding for doctors, nurses, and dieticians attending to the prevention of and care for the obese (House of Commons Health Committee, 2016, p. 23). Notwithstanding these budget cuts, the Conservative–Liberal Democrat Coalition government essentially continued the strategy pursued by New Labour, though with renewed faith in the ability of behavioural techniques to control obesity.

The new *Call to Action on Obesity*, launched in November 2011, reiterated the need for changes to individual behaviour while recognizing that the environment is important for enabling individuals to choose a healthy lifestyle. The Coalition government emphasized that it 'favours interventions towards the less intrusive end of the Nuffield ladder – with a focus on equipping people to make the best possible choices' (Department of Health, 2011, p. 6). Nevertheless, like New Labour, the Coalition government maintained the need for concerted and extensive interventions by central government, local authorities, and various private actors to support individuals in adopting healthier lifestyles (Department of Health, 2011, pp. 7–8).

Like the wider health promotion policies, obesity control under the two recent Conservative-led governments has oscillated between rational choice and behavioural strategies, both targeting individuals. The rational strategy, which assumes the existence of a responsible individual making more healthy decisions as he or she grows more enlightened, was articulated in the *2010 to 2015 Government Policy: Obesity and Healthy Eating* (Department of Health, 2015a). Here the strategy of '[h]elping people to make healthier choices' was principally to be achieved by giving people advice and guidance and improving food labelling so that they can make healthy choices. In line with the widespread public budget cuts launched by the Coalition government, the rational choice health strategy entailed launching the Public Health Responsibility Deal (PHRD) in 2011. This was to replace government funding for the Change4Life programme, which had been launched by New Labour in 2009. This programme included, among other things, the '10 minutes shake-up' campaign targeting children, a joint venture between Public Health England and Disney (Public Health England, 2014, p. 14). While Change4Life has continued, it was increasingly financed by for-profit and non-profit organizations. It has been duly noted that what 'is good for income generation of sponsors and supporters, is not necessarily good for health' (Ulijaszek and McLennan, 2016, p. 406).

Interestingly, neither New Labour nor the Conservative Party has shown much interest in using economic incentives to change people's lifestyle. Of course, the fear of being accused of wanting to embark on big government and increase public spending is likely to go quite some way in explaining this reluctance. Informed by a medical report suggesting an increase of at least 20 per cent in soft drink duty as an experimental pilot to learn more about the behavioural effects (Royal College of Paediatrics and Child Health, 2015, p. 5), the Conservative government announced – in its *Childhood Obesity: A Plan for Action* (HM Government, 2016) – the introduction (from 2018) of a 20 per cent levy on soft drinks, i.e. a tax targeting the producers rather than the consumers. The remainder of this action plan, which has been heavily criticized by health experts and local authorities for its lack of regulations and investments (O'Dowd, 2016), included assisting the food industry in reducing sugar contents in and providing clearer information about their products, encouraging state schools to offer more physical activity and healthier food, and monitoring their progress on this.

If neither New Labour nor the Conservatives have shown much interest in employing rational actor strategies and economic incentives to control obesity, they seem to have great hopes for behavioural approaches, notably nudging, to control obesity, which has attracted much more government interest. The Department of Health report, *Living Well for Longer: One Year On* aimed to 'stimulate a focus on creating and protecting health, not only treating ill-health; identifying the opportunities for tackling the major public health issues using evidence including behavioural sciences' (Department of Health, 2015b, p. 12). Instead of working (only) through the responsible and rational individual, the strategy outlined in *Living Well for Longer* was trying to pave the way for interventions that would make individuals change their behaviour by latching on to and directing their unconscious drives and predispositions. Parts of these changes are firstly about modifying the (urban) physical environment to make physical exercise an easier choice. This may include developing new or existing park areas, creating bike lanes, introducing cycle parking, dropping pavement kerbs, adding showers at workplaces, or improving stairwells (Public Health England, 2014, p. 17). Secondly, other changes seek to modify the unconscious choices people make by, for example, having arrows on the floor pointing to the nearest staircase (rather than the elevator). The Social Marketing Unit established under the auspices of the Department of Health in 2004 aimed to make the way that authorities communicate with the public more effective by using insights from behavioural psychology (Jones et al., 2013, p. 116). However, so far, the main strategy pursued by the Social Marketing Unit has been to make use of social media to convey traditional messages about the importance of diet and exercise (Public Health England, 2015a, pp. 14–15, 34–35). The most innovative measures informed by behavioural psychology seem to be the fine-tuning of search engine algorithms, which would make it easier to search the internet for obesity control advice, and to make supermarkets remove sweets from the exit (Public Health England, 2015a, p. 32), a location originally recommended by behavioural psychologists employed by supermarkets to boost the sales of sweets! Thirdly, based on the psychological assumption that many people get discouraged partly by the many – often conflicting – experts providing advice and partly by the magnitude of the time and effort required to change their everyday life and lose weight, the British Nutrition Foundation launched the Small Changes, Big Gains campaign in 2012 (British Nutrition Foundation, 2012). For example, it urges people to set minor, realistic targets of exercise (e.g. ten minutes per day) and keep a record of their progress towards these goals. In sum, behavioural psychology has inspired a number of minor initiatives seeking to make people change their diet and exercise more in order to lose weight. However, in spite of much fanfare about the potential of behaviourist approaches, the number and scope of techniques employed in the area of obesity control still seem rather limited.

The two individualizing approaches explored above do not stand alone but are complemented by a renewed focus on the health promoting potential of communities. Under the Health and Social Care Act 2012, local governments (municipalities) were charged with the responsibility for monitoring the health and wellbeing status of local communities and designing integrated strategies seeking to improve this status (Health and Social Care Act 2012, part 5, ch. 2). The Coalition government regarded local governments as being in a favourable position both to meet the different needs of their specific communities and to make diverse individuals and groups and public and private actors join forces to improve health. In an attempt to reinvigorate the – constantly failing – attempt to reduce the number of obese people, the NHS launched a series of new interventions as part of its *Five Years Forward View* in October 2014 (NHS England, 2014a). In a speech made shortly prior to the launch, NHS director Simon Stevens cited the fact that one in five secondary schoolchildren is now obese and warned that:

> Unchecked, the result will inevitably be a huge rise in avoidable illness and disability, including many cases of type 2 diabetes which Diabetes UK estimate already costs the NHS around £9 billion a year … Obesity is the new smoking, and it represents a slow-motion car crash in terms of avoidable illness and rising health care costs … If as a nation we keep piling on the pounds around the waistline, we'll be piling on the pounds in terms of future taxes needed just to keep the NHS afloat. (NHS England, 2014b)

The *Five Year Forward View* strategy essentially amounts to more of the same, i.e. the pursuit of a rather narrow focus on prevention and health promotion in the fight against obesity. Without any further documentation, it is argued that preventive approaches to obesity are preferable to bariatric surgery and, consequently, the latter should be reduced in favour of a nationwide prevention programme targeting obesity and diabetes (NHS England, 2014a, p. 11). Local government, communities, and workplaces are envisaged to play an important role in preventing obesity and promoting health. For example, local government may prohibit the establishment of outlets for junk food close to schools, voluntary organizations and individuals should provide advice to local citizens, and employers should be provided with incentives to encourage employees to engage in vocational rehabilitation.

Local governments have embraced the strategy, in which they play a crucial role in obesity control. As explained by the Local Government Association:

> Councils are the best placed public sector organisations to lead on tackling overweight before it becomes a problem, joining up services with leisure centres, transport, education about health and community-run activity schemes. (Local Government Association, 2015, p. 9)

Citing the Foresight analysis' recommendation to pursue a multi-pronged approach targeting biological, environmental, psychological, social, physical, and other factors, the Local Government Association proposed that parts of the money generated by raising VAT on sweets and sugary drinks and the duty on tobacco could be used by local councils to finance a wide range of obesity control interventions. These interventions could include increasing cycling and walking routes, supporting or establishing farmers' markets and other initiatives securing the availability of affordable and healthy food stuffs in deprived areas, or working with school teachers to improve education in cooking healthy food (Local Government Association, 2015, pp. 11–13). The interventions would also include establishing local, multi-professional centres to provide advice for the obese, making GPs work with local employers on how they can contribute to better diet and more exercise at work, supporting local sports clubs to mobilize more people to be physically active, and working with day care providers and nurseries to improve the diet and physical development of children. The list of initiatives used to mobilize local actors and institutions to create a dense web of mechanisms in support of making citizens adopt a better diet and engage in regular physical exercise seems endless. The main barrier for knitting together this web seems to be the permanent lack of adequate public funding (Local Government Association, 2015, p. 10).

In sum, the Cameron-led Coalition government pursued obesity control using a strategy that essentially emulates that of New Labour. Political emphasis has been not only or even primarily on the two individualizing strategies (rational choice and behavioural techniques) but also on attempts to create an enabling environment by making local government, communities, and employers aid in the fight against obesity. If there is any political or medical critique of this preventive strategy working through local public and private organizations, it has to do with complaints about the inadequate funding and regulations enabling the conduct of healthier lifestyles (House of Commons Health Committee, 2016). Few if any seem to debate whether this strategy is politically desirable and/or economically cost-effective.

Governing for a healthy future: individualizing techniques targeting children

Child obesity has caused particular concern among medical scientists and public health authorities. If obesity in general constitutes an important and growing health and financial concern, child obesity is regarded as particularly problematic by changing English governments and their health authorities. The reason is that obesity in childhood is widely regarded as increasing the likelihood of obesity later in life. Accordingly, the health problems and the public fiscal costs linked to treating these problems are likely to increase substantially if left unchecked. Thus, for the sake both of the citizen and the (control of) public health expenditures, British health authorities have devoted particular attention to the question of how to control childhood obesity over the last two decades or so. Just how strong the political importance attributed to fighting childhood obesity is may be indicated by several incidences of forced removal of children from their parents on the grounds that they did not take adequate care of their children's health, including controlling obesity. A 2007 BBC survey reported that obesity had played a role in at least 20 child protection cases in the previous year (Viner, Roche, Maguire, and Nicholls, 2010, p. 375). However, the use of coercion in obesity control in England is rare and, as should be clear from the following, an exception to the general pattern of governing through the freedom of children and their parents.

The National Child Measurement Programme (NCMP) was established in 2005/06 with the task of gathering population-level data to allow for analysis of trends in growth patterns and obesity (Public Health England, 2015b). These data are to be used at a national level to support local public health initiatives and inform the local planning and delivery of services for children. NCMP measures the height and weight of children in reception class (aged 4 to 5 years) and Year 6 (aged 10 to 11 years) to assess overweight and obesity levels in children within primary schools. The measurement process is overseen by trained healthcare professionals in schools. Every year, more than 1 million children are measured and over 99.5 per cent of eligible schools take part on a voluntary basis. Children's heights and weights are measured and used to calculate a BMI centile. The individualizing data on child weight is used as the basis for parents, schools, and local health authorities to target overweight and obese children. After each round of measuring, parents receive a letter reporting on the weight of their child, whether the result means that the child is underweight, normal, or overweight, and providing information on how to get further advice on diet and exercise for children (National Child Measurement Programme, 2015). The data are collected by the Health and Social Care Information Centre and are not disclosed to anyone except the child's parents. However, recently an expert paediatric report explicitly recommended that researchers and clinicians (including the family GP and the relevant school nurse) be allowed to access the data (Royal College of Paediatrics and Child Health, 2015, p. 5).

The decision on whether to take action on the basis of the NCMP data rests with the parents of the child. Yet this does not mean that the data are not used by others besides the parents to suggest action. Schools and public health nurses play an important role in providing advice to overweight children and their parents on diet and physical exercise (Davies, Gardner, and White, 2015). While the nurses have access to NCMP data only at the school level, not at the level of the individual pupil, the NCMP data are conducive to the follow-up work by the nurses in at least two ways. First of all, the nurse will be made aware if a particular school is showing high levels of obesity frequency compared to other schools in Britain. Secondly, the fact that parents of overweight/obese children receive an authoritative letter from the Health and Social Information Centre stating that their child has a weight problem is likely to make it easier for the nurse to convince the parents that their child has a problem and that they should take action. This is relevant, as some ethnic groups seem less inclined to believe that their child has a weight problem despite the NCMP showing the opposite (Davies et al., 2015). More generally, the school nurses are envisaged to play a key role in the health of schoolchildren during all stages of their stay at school (Public Health England et al., 2014). Together with local community organizations, health services, the GP, and other relevant organizations, the nurse is supposed to act both as a driver and as a relay for identifying and taking actions targeting overweight children. These actions include promoting a healthy diet and lifestyle, promoting physical activity, discussing emotional health and wellbeing (recognizing that obesity may be related to low self-esteem), promoting school routine/avoiding truancy, and involving parents and the wider family.

Of course, we should be careful not to exaggerate the influence of school nurse interventions in the lives of schoolchildren. Thus, the ongoing public sector budget cuts launched by the Cameron government seem to have effectively reduced the capacity to undertake effective work by school nurses in the area of obesity control (*Guardian*, 2015). However, in our view, the rationale of these budget cuts does not express any fundamental break with the will to fight child obesity through preventive and health promotion strategies. For example, in 2013 local governments were charged with the responsibility for delivering the National Child Measurement Programme (Local Government Association, 2013). This programme, which has run since 2006, was to be reinvigorated by making local governments adopt a 'joined-up' approach that would involve paying attention to children's ideas and creating networks of health community champions (health trainers, school canteen staff, youth club leaders). The programme also urged local governments to cooperate with other public agencies (planning, transport, education, and leisure) and private actors (workplace canteens and restaurants) through, for example, healthy eating award schemes (Local Government Association, 2013, p. 6). Thus, while the budget cuts conducted from 2010 onwards most likely have impeded the realization of policy goals to reduce the prevalence of obesity, the budget cuts have not terminated the will to intervene in the daily life of obese children and young people.

This will to control child obesity by health promotion seems to remain the crux of government health politics, a will that may be illustrated by the flourishing of overweight camps. These camps constitute a relatively recent but increasingly popular health intervention. Such camps have been run by private (for-profit) organizations and more recently by the NHS. Some of the first weight loss camps were the Carnegie International Camps, organized in the early 1990s under the auspices of Professor Paul Gately and his colleagues from Leeds Metropolitan University (MoreLife, 2016). After visits to similar camps in the US, they found these not to be very effective because of a rather narrow focus on diet and physical exercise. The US camps overlooked social psychological factors or, more precisely, the role played by self-esteem and peer relations. Subsequently, the obesity research group from Leeds Metropolitan University went to some lengths to demonstrate the relationship between psychological factors and being overweight (Gately, Cooke, Butterly, Mackreath, and Carroll, 2000; L. Walker, Gately, Bewick, and Hill, 2003). While researchers in this field remain cautious about the direction of causality, the programmes informed by this research clearly see low self-esteem and peer relations as a contributing factor to being overweight. Hence, there is a need for a number of 'social' activities that will help children and young people improve their self-esteem and peer relations, and thereby their capacity to develop and maintain a healthy lifestyle.

Directly inspired by the Carnegie International Camps, the NHS has sponsored annual overweight camps run by various organizations. For example, the privately run FitFarms have since 2006 catered both to paying clients and to children paid for by the NHS (FitFarms, 2016). In order to ensure sustainable changes in lifestyle, a key element in the weight-loss approach adopted at FitFarms is enabling the participants to make individualized programmes that best suit their needs and desires. Another famous example is the Rotherham camp, which has operated since 2008 (NHS Rotherham, 2010). Located in an area with a very high incidence of overweight people – among both adults and children – the Rotherham camp has been supported to offer services both to adults and to children with severe weight problems. At Rotherham, children and young persons are placed in a structured exercise and lifestyle programme, though 'with the emphasis on having fun' (NHS Rotherham, 2010). The mainstay of the course is: physical activity, diet, lifestyle education, and social activity. Physical activities typically include six hours per day including running, karate, basketball, and team games. With regard to diet habits, the children were taught about nutrition, the importance of a balanced diet, portion sizes, and having everyday food in moderation. In particular, they were instructed on how to make healthy food. Moreover, inspired by the Carnegie International Camp approach, in which social activities are seen as helpful for building self-esteem, which in turn is regarded as beneficial to build a durable healthy lifestyle, all children participate in social activities, such as discos, day trips, and talent nights as well as hobby-type clubs including photography and performing arts. In very prosaic terms, to lose fat, kids must have fun (NHS Rotherham, 2010). Thus, we see a form of governmental power working by directing kids to freely subject themselves as psychological subjects of self-esteem. Rather than exercising power in the form of an externally imposed disciplinary regimen of diet and physical activity, inn this example the children must learn to look into themselves to find and mobilize their resources both individually and, in particular, in groups with other children. Finally, parents and families are involved through meetings held before, during, and after the camp in order to create an environment conducive to the children's choice of a healthy lifestyle after the camp.

Until recently, occasional tabloid articles suggested that the NHS was relatively restrictive in allowing overweight children to access the camps, which are fairly expensive (M. Evans, 2014). However, more recently, the NHS decided to expand the number of these camps and the persons admitted to them in order to fight type 2 diabetes (NHS England, 2016). Thus, in 2016 the programme, which caters to both children and adults, was rolled out in 27 areas and made up to 20,000 places available. By 2020, it is expected that the programme will cover the whole country and make 100,000 referrals available each year. In brief, it seems that the fit (or fat) camps constitute an increasingly important technique for controlling obesity by way of individualizing techniques bolstering the self-esteem and practical skills of children and, to a lesser extent, adults.

Conclusion

This chapter has shown that obesity control had already emerged in the early twentieth century, i.e. well before neoliberal rationalities began informing public health interventions in England. At that time, the focus was on obesity as a sign of the degeneration of the British race. After a long interlude, obesity was rearticulated as a political problem in the 1980s, when medical evidence pointed to its relationship to cardiac diseases, various forms of cancer, and diabetes. While a preventive and integrated approach was suggested, very little concerted action was taken until the late 1990s. The main intervention took the form of improved information (product labelling and information campaigns) in order to appeal to the rational and responsible liberal subject.

From the late 1990s, the community became a key site of intervention for the fight against obesity. It was imagined that community empowerment – in various forms – would strengthen the possibilities for citizens to choose a healthy lifestyle. This neoliberal (constructivist) strategy has, with some variations, remained the dominant one until today. So far, individualizing strategies have played a more limited role, though several techniques have been developed targeting the obese. One of the most spectacular techniques is the so-called fat camps where obese children and – in increasingly more cases – adults are trained in the art of governing themselves in a healthy manner. Here the focus is not only on dieting and physical exercise but also on social activities, in order to develop the self-esteem of the obese. While there has been much talk during the 2010s on the potential of nudging techniques, this has played a rather limited role so far, mostly due to practical problems with adopting viable solutions. Thus, the relatively limited spread of nudging and community empowerment seems to have less to do with classical liberal concerns over excessive state intervention and more to do with concerns over public expenditures and technical difficulties in making empowerment and nudging work in the area of obesity control.

At the most general level, the chapter has shown the development of a quite comprehensive apparatus of central and local authorities teaming up with voluntary organizations and for-profit organizations to govern in the name of the community. This apparatus has in many ways failed when judged by its own terms, i.e. the reduction of obesity in England. Yet it has succeeded in the sense that the persistence of obesity has resulted in calls for more interventions to empower communities and their citizens, rather than fewer. Thus, changing English governments since the late 1990s have relied not only on appeals to the rational citizen by way of product labelling and information campaigns but also on direct interventions targeting the communities and individual obese persons. The contemporary obesity apparatus does seem to be expanding and seemingly limitless, not only because it identifies and targets 'patients before their time' (B. Evans and Colls, 2011) but also because its failure is used as an argument for the need for its expansion. The homology with Foucault's analysis of the disciplinary and rehabilitating strategy informing prison reforms in the early nineteenth century seems obvious (Foucault, 1977).

At a more specific level, this apparently unlimited quest to try and control obesity has more to do with contemporary constructivist neoliberalism than with the kind of early nineteenth-century forms of disciplinary power that Foucault analysed. What current British public health programmes are trying to do is not so much to discipline individuals as to empower them, i.e. to make them exercise their freedom in a way that will promote their health. We also find that contemporary

English obesity management may be understood in terms of optimistic vitalism in the sense that there seems to be no limit to just how healthy the English citizen has to be before she is outside the scope of obesity control programmes. Of course, we should be very careful not to exaggerate the implications of this quest. As we shall see in the following chapter on obesity control in Denmark, the English programmes are less well organized, seem to receive less funding, and, obviously, are not very successful in meeting their own objective (making the English population less overweight).

Note

1 The 'whole-population' approach was a feature of a WHO report, *Prevention of Coronary Heart Disease*, published the previous year (WHO, 1982).

4
Governing obesity in Denmark

Over the last two decades, obesity has become a major political concern in Denmark. In tandem with the growing numbers of overweight and obese individuals, epidemiologists, doctors, health economists, social workers, and politicians have in various ways problematized obesity and articulated the need for systematic intervention. While there are substantial debates and disagreements about how best to tackle the problem of obesity, there are few who dispute the need for political interventions in the area. There is a sense of urgency: if public authorities and private actors do not engage in concerted action against obesity, the general health of the Danish population will deteriorate and a number of specific diseases (such as diabetes, cardiovascular diseases, and certain forms of cancer) will proliferate – as will the public expenditures for treating these diseases. Many citizens will lead an impoverished life and will lose their attachment to the labour market, with a negative impact on the entire Danish economy. This is, broadly speaking, the problematization that informs the debates and disputes: not whether political action is needed, but how it should be done.

In the midst of this general problematization, we do find a few critical voices addressing the norms and power engaged in the fight against obesity. In particular, the Danish anthropologist Nanna Mik-Meyer has critically examined the contemporary fight against obesity and the moral imperatives that are being imposed on individual citizens on how to lead their lives. Both the schemes unfolding in specific (public and private) workplaces and the more general health promotion interventions rest, she argues, on a particular constellation of biomedical norms about the ideal physical body (based on body mass index (BMI) and other indicators) on the one hand and social values about self-control on the other hand (Mik-Meyer, 2008, 2014). This constellation amounts to a rather narrow understanding of a responsible lifestyle, which is imposed on school pupils, employees, and citizens in general. While the imposition of these values takes place by non-coercive means, the individuals who do not subject themselves to these values are regarded as morally inferior and irresponsible (Mik-Meyer, 2010). We largely agree with this critique of obesity interventions, which has also been articulated by other scholars outside Denmark (e.g. Jutel, 2005; Murray, 2005).

This chapter seeks to take the critique of obesity interventions in Denmark a step further by trying to better understand how the kind of moral values and power ingrained in the current fight against power became the obvious choice. Put differently, how and why there has been so little debate about health promotion interventions? This is odd considering that the current fight against obesity shows few inhibitions in terms of intervening more or less directly in the lives of every citizen, not only the sick and not only those deemed at risk. To get a better understanding of this, we need to examine in some detail the historical emergence of the kinds of knowledge, problematizations, and particular kinds of power making up health promotion in the area of obesity control. Our general argument is that the epidemiological and welfare economic objectification and problematization of obesity rendered political action both possible and necessary, in the sense that it would be seen as irresponsible for any politician to do nothing. Moreover, the emphasis on health promotion, which is based on an indirect form of power that works through the free subjection of citizens, made it difficult to articulate any protest against these interventions, even if the norms of healthy conduct or lifestyle are narrow and potentially stigmatize a range of other lifestyles.

This chapter examines how obesity became of the object of biomedical and political concern through epidemiological studies. Moreover, it accounts for the key health promotion programmes employed to control obesity in Denmark. Finally, the chapter examines the working of health promotion by exploring two concrete obesity control programmes.

Historical antecedents

The current concern over obesity in the Danish population may have reached unprecedented levels in the last two decades or so, but it is not an entirely new phenomenon. As part of a generalized concern about the quality of the Danish stock during the 1920s and 1930s, people's weight received substantial attention from medical experts and laymen. By the same token, a medical-cum-popular movement arose under the name of constructive hygiene or positive eugenics, with the aim of ensuring the mental, moral, and physical quality of the Danish population.

As in England, the main concern was with underweight individuals resulting from under- or malnutrition. In particular, there was a strong concern over undernourished children among the poor classes, as it was envisaged that they would fall prey to a number of diseases later in life, such as tuberculosis, and therefore that their labour power and contribution to society would be reduced. However, in contrast to the present-day attempts to control obesity, Danish health authorities played a very minor role in this field during the 1920s and 1930s. Equipped with new biometric measuring methods, a new profession of nurses or health visitors would seek out and visit poor families and schools to examine the weight and general health of children and, if necessary, take steps to ensure that they received a better diet (Vucina, 2014, pp. 127–128). As we shall see in this chapter, this intrusion into the lives of children and youth via their families and schools is repeated today. A host of nurses, health assistants, and social workers, equipped with new biometric measuring standards and techniques, such as BMI, are singling out the obese or, even better, those deemed at risk of becoming obese.

Being underweight no doubt constituted the most important political concern in terms of people's weight at the beginning of the twentieth century. Yet being overweight was a concern for public authorities and others, too. As in England, the deteriorating influence of the various forms of sedentary work occupying an increasing proportion of Danes' employment was problematized both by health authorities and by a number of gymnastic pedagogues (Bonde, 1991, pp. 165–178). The concern over obesity was linked to the wider question of how to ensure the wellbeing and welfare of the Danish population, an increasingly important question during the 1920s and 1930s. With the Social Democrats as the lead, all the major Danish political parties were concerned about how to be able to afford to provide health, education, and social services for a growing population with a view towards alleviating poor health, illiteracy, and poverty. One of the answers to this question was the simultaneous emergence of eugenics and the welfare economy. In particular, the ideas fostered by the Swedish couple Alva and Gunnar Myrdal about the need to control the procreation of the mentally and physically ill in order to be able to afford and ensure the welfare of the wider population were particularly influential (Myrdal and Myrdal, 1935; Kemp, 1937). An intense debate ensued from the late 1920s to the mid-1930s over the potential and acceptability of negative eugenics. While all political parties rejected elimination, there was a strong support for prevention, i.e. attempts to hinder the procreation of inferior individuals (Koch, 2000). This evolved into laws that allowed sterilization of the feeble-minded. This would eventually include individuals with a variety of mental health diagnoses, alcoholics, and prostitutes. Even if the law required the consent of the individual, more than 60,000 people were sterilized over the next three decades.

If political authorities were deeply engaged in negative eugenics, they played a limited role in positive eugenics or constructive hygiene, as it was also called at the time (Munck, 1935). During the early twentieth century, gymnastics and sports organizations were established all over Denmark. These were private organizations, though they often received some level of financial support from the state. Informed partly by nation-building concerns and partly by concerns over the fear of 'feminization' of males increasingly occupied in sedentary and monotonous work in offices and factories, the gymnastics and sports organizations aspired to promote bodily culture and development among the entire Danish population (Bonde, 1991; Vucina, 2014, p. 135). More precisely, they envisaged that regular physical training of the body would not only cure physical weakness (obesity), but it would also cure mental weakness by strengthening the person's moral character. Gymnastics was seen as a moral weapon against indolence, dullness, and indulgence. Supported by medical experts, general practitioners, nurses, gymnastics pedagogues, and a number of self-taught individuals, gymnastics was propagated not only in the growing gymnastics and sports organizations but also at schools and in private homes. In order to instil in children the importance of physical exercise, gymnastics had been a compulsory part of the (elementary) public school curriculum since the early nineteenth century. However, it was only in 1904, following mounting critiques from pedagogues and army officers, that the content of the gymnastics lessons became subject to state regulation and monitoring (Jørgensen, 1998, p. 85). This reform was linked to the highly popular ideas and techniques espoused by Jørgen Peter Müller, a former army lieutenant, a highly proficient athlete, and an inspector at one of the largest tuberculosis sanatoriums in Denmark. In 1903, Müller won a beauty contest for men, and the following year he published the book *My System* (*Mit system*), which was subsequently translated into 25 languages and printed in more than 1.5 million copies (Müller, 1904; Ettrup and Olsen, 2014). Moreover, the advent of national radio, which spread to most Danish households during the 1930s, allowed a number of highly popular, self-taught individuals, such as Captain Jespersen, to reach Danes in their own homes and teach them how to perform basic physical exercises every day (Vucina, 2014, p. 137).

The fight against obesity during the 1920s and 1930s took place almost exclusively through individualizing interventions that, in turn, were predominantly propagated by private organizations, medical experts, and self-taught individuals. The main role of the state was to make nurses inspect the health of children shortly after birth and at school and to adopt regulations making gymnastics part of the school syllabus. Similarly, external, environmental interventions played a very limited role, if any, in weight control. Thus, the widespread introduction of clean water, sewage systems, waste management, building regulations, and hygienic standards for food processing, which were launched from the end of the nineteenth century up to the 1940s, were aimed at preventing the spread of disease and raising the general health level of the population. They did not aim at addressing concrete problems like unhealthy diet or inadequate physical exercise. This relatively restrictive role of both the state and the environmental interventions is remarkable not only because malnourishment and inadequate physical exercise were seen as serious problems in the early twentieth century but also because both the state and environmental interventions would come to play a crucial role from the 1990s onwards in controlling obesity.

In conceptual terms, the (public and private) interventions targeting obesity at that time were informed by a mix of social welfarist (including eugenic) and liberal rationales. On the one hand, these interventions aimed at promoting public wellbeing by a number of more or less direct interventions targeting the individual. On the other hand, concerns over the integrity of the individual and over expenditure in the area of public health limited these interventions.

Objectifying obesity

Since the early 1990s, a number of epidemiological surveys have illuminated and problematized the phenomenon of obesity in the Danish population.[1] Above all, the surveys conducted by the Danish Institute for Clinical Epidemiology, which changed its name in 1999 to the State Institute for Public Health, have since the early 1990s made extensive and systematic studies of the national prevalence of obesity in Denmark. In line with international biomedical standards in the field, BMI has played a crucial role in the Danish attempts to objectify and quantify the phenomenon of obesity.

Together with BMI, the unique Danish central person-registration system enabled the production of extensive and precise epidemiological studies of the prevalence of obesity. For example, in 2010 and 2013, the State Institute of Public Health issued a very detailed national health profile study correlating obesity with a number of geographic, demographic, and socioeconomic variables (Statens Institut for Folkesundhed, 2013). These studies inform state, regional, and municipal obesity control interventions not only by visualizing and problematizing obesity but also by pinpointing the correlations between obesity on the one hand, and municipal residence, occupation, education, marital status, age, and gender on the other. Apart from these national studies, we also find minor surveys. The Database for Children's Health (Databasen Børns Sundhed), for example, is a joint project between 13 municipalities in greater Copenhagen that was established in 2002 in order to monitor children's health and the municipal health services and to provide a basis for the development of the latter (Statens Institut for Folkesundhed, 2016). The Database for Children's Health is updated annually with basic health information, including obesity, of children from 0 to 1 year and at 6 years of age. It has been used both by health researchers and by politicians to assess the utility of the municipalities' many initiatives to fight obesity launched since the mid-2000s (Kudahl, 2012). By and large, the statistics are taken to indicate that the municipal initiatives launched over the last decade have contributed to reducing obesity rates but that the existing efforts must be consolidated.

Moreover, the craze for evidence-based policymaking has also found its way into contemporary Danish obesity control. Thus, we find a number of expert reports assessing the effectiveness of the growing number of interventions targeting the obese. For example, the former Danish Hospital Institute (DSI) and the current Danish Institute for Local and Regional Government Research are directly focusing on providing evidence for the efficacy of various health interventions, including those targeting obesity and lifestyle changes (e.g. E. Hansen, 2012; Martin and Nielsen, 2012; Jansbøl and Rahbek, 2013). These publications tend to conclude that a comprehensive approach targeting diet, physical exercise, and behavioural competences, on the one hand, and the immediate environment of the obese, such as parents in the case of obese children, on the other hand, seems to be most effective. In brief, a combination of extensive epidemiological knowledge has emerged with the effect of illuminating and framing obesity as a problem of the national population's biological quality and longevity. Since the mid-2000s this knowledge has become increasingly detailed and focused around the correlation between obesity and a range of environmental variables. More recently, a second body of policy evaluation knowledge has emerged with a view towards rendering the problem of obesity amenable to government intervention and, more precisely, stimulating and legitimizing further interventions by assessing their efficacy.

Finally, we find local assessments based on less tangible, *savoir-faire*-based notions of risk. BMI has proved a useful standard in gauging the national prevalence of obesity. Yet it is deemed of little use for identifying those at risk of becoming obese. Because health promotion is not satisfied with identifying and curing those regarded as obese but insists on preventing the emergence of obesity, two other indicators have played a certain role in Danish obesity control, namely waist measurements and instances of family members being overweight. Firstly, health nurses, health assistants, social workers, and other welfare state engineers employed in contemporary obesity control have noticed that many children and young person with a normal BMI still display above-average waist measurements. Such young people are sometimes referred to as 'thin-fat' kids, and health nurses have expressed concern over many children and young persons who may not be overweight but who display underdeveloped muscular structure and at the same time too much fat around their waistline. According to the *savoir-faire* of the health nurses, these bodily signs are often an indication of a sedentary lifestyle that eventually may lead to being overweight or obese. Consequently, such signs should be and are, to some extent, taken into consideration when singling out children in need of assistance. Secondly, children and young persons with overweight or obese siblings or parents are regarded as being at high risk of becoming obese. Even if the child has a normal BMI and is not seen as 'thin-fat', the prevailing assumption is that the diet and physical habits of the family are very likely to influence those of the child (Vucina, 2014, pp. 157–158). Again, this calls for concern and early detection in order to discourage the child from adopting the problematic health behaviour of her family.

In sum, we find a wide range of quite distinct forms of knowledge production enabling and structuring obesity control. These include at least two forms of highly scientific forms of knowledge, namely epidemiological, register-based surveys gauging the prevalence of obesity and experimental trials gauging the effect of various policy instruments. Both these have been highly influential is gauging and visualizing the problem of obesity and in finding and examining ways of handling this problem. Yet we also find less formalized and, some would say, less scientific forms of knowledge, namely the waist measurements and weight of the child's family. Later in this chapter, we shall see how these more mundane forms of knowledge inform the everyday work of obesity control.

Governing obesity: enter the public authorities

As we showed at the beginning of this chapter, concerns over obesity among the Danish population can be dated at least back to the 1920s. However, this concern resulted in relatively limited interventions by public authorities revolving around gymnastics in the public school. With the systematic epidemiological accounts of the proliferation of obesity during the 1990s and the medical linking of obesity to cardiovascular diseases, diabetes, several forms of cancer, and other diseases, public authorities gradually began to use their powers to try to control obesity.

The first attempt to systematize the fight against obesity came in early 2003 with the Danish Health Authority's *Proposal for a National Action Plan against Severe Obesity – Proposals for Solutions and Perspectives* (Sundhedsstyrelsen, 2003). The action plan was strongly supported by the Danish Society for Obesity Research, which had committed itself – via its interactions with the WHO Milan Declaration – to the making of a national strategy (Svendsen et al., 2001, p. 3). The Danish Society for Obesity Research recommended, in line with the WHO, pursuing interventions targeting those citizens already suffering from obesity and interventions aimed at general prevention, i.e. the whole population (Svendsen et al., 2001, pp. 8–9). The Danish Health Authority's action plan had a broad scope too, though its strategy remained somewhat unclear. Thus, it contained a stunning 66 recommendations targeting three sectors of society: the private level (the individual citizen, the family, and their immediate environment), communities (schools, workplaces, and voluntary organizations), and the public level (state, counties, and municipalities). In line with the wider health promotion strategy, it was emphasized that the control of obesity required a joint effort across the whole of society.

The Health Authority's action plan was followed in the period 2005 to 2008 by the allocation of 7 million DKK to 26 one-year projects seeking to control obesity (Sundhedsstyrelsen, 2012a). The projects were run by hospitals, municipal health care services, specialized social care institutions, private gymnastics associations, and universities. The target groups ranged from pregnant women and schoolchildren to adults living in poor urban areas who all suffered from various levels of obesity. The short-term nature of these projects notwithstanding, the Health Authority concluded that the fight against obesity requires long-term interventions that involve cooperation between a wide range of public and private actors (Sundhedsstyrelsen, 2012a, p. 4). A few other projects were inaugurated around 2003 and 2004 such as Everything about Diet – Taste for Life, a project seeking to encourage schools and kindergartens to provide healthy meals for children. Another project, Health Sign, which included schools, kindergartens, day care centres, and sports clubs, aimed at encouraging children to make healthy food, exercise, not smoking, and good hygiene a part of their everyday life (Indenrigs- og Sundhedsministeriet, 2005, p. 10).

A second series of projects targeting the obesity of children and young persons was conducted between 2005 and 2008 (Sundhedsstyrelsen, 2012e). These projects, which were run by more than 30 municipalities, all had two target levels: *the individuals* suffering from obesity (focusing on improving their self-esteem, physical activity, and healthy diet) and *the environment* of all children and young people (focusing on providing environments in schools and various youth clubs conducive to physical exercise and healthy eating). Finally, a few generalized interventions targeting the whole population were launched, notably the updating and dissemination of national dietary guidelines, which were widely broadcast on national television, and new health labelling of the most common food products indicating their fat and sugar content (Sundhedsstyrelsen, 2012e, p. 14).

Stepping up municipal health promotion interventions

The ambition of the 2003 Health Authority action plan to systematize the many initiatives launched to regulate obesity notwithstanding, these projects remained somewhat unsystematic and their scope mostly limited. It is only with the structural reform of 2007, whereby the municipalities were charged with the task of health promotion, that obesity slowly but steadily became an object of systematic and comprehensive political intervention. Following a period of uncertainty about the new role of the municipalities after the structural reform, they gradually embarked on interventions targeting not only obese individuals but also the general environment that may lead to or (preferably) prevent obesity. In order to try to assist and systematize the municipalities' health promotion efforts, the Health Authority launched the Prevention Package for Obesity (Sundhedsstyrelsen, 2013). Like the other health promotion packages mentioned above, this one provided an overview of the prevalence of obesity, its economic costs, the evidence for the efficacy of various interventions, and an overview of some of the many municipal initiatives launched so far. Again, the Health Authority insisted that the fight against obesity required not only that municipal employees at all levels have a thorough knowledge of relevant and effective lifestyle interventions but also that they engage in cooperation and partnerships with a wide range of relevant actors, such as schools, parents, youth and sports clubs, workplaces, and general practitioners (Sundhedsstyrelsen, 2013, p. 29).

But how far have the 98 Danish municipalities gone in developing and implementing health promotion initiatives? This is a really difficult question to answer. An evaluation of the municipalities' activities between 2013 and 2014 showed that 44 per cent of all municipalities had developed obesity-control services targeting the entire family, and 71 per cent had developed initiatives targeting schoolchildren (N. Christiansen et al., 2014). The following year, the latter figure rose to 74 per cent (N. Christiansen, Holmberg, Hærvig, Christensen, and Rod, 2015, p. 85). In the following, we try to sketch out what we have found to be the most important initiatives. Yet it should be stressed that we do not try to give a precise account of just how far each of these types of interventions have developed in each of the 98 municipalities.

At the most general level, municipalities have initiated five types of programmes or procedures for tackling obesity since 2007. All five types are encouraged by the Danish Health Authority (Sundhedsstyrelsen,

2013). Firstly, the Danish Health Authority has urged all 98 municipalities to develop specific *policies and action plans* for fighting obesity (Sundhedsstyrelsen, 2013, p. 19). The policies should include quantifiable targets for reducing the number of citizens suffering from obesity. They also include the development of concrete services, information, education, and early tracing of citizens at risk of obesity. Finally, such plans should work across organizational boundaries within the municipality and together with relevant organizations, such as schools, sports associations, and workplaces. While most, if not all, municipalities have developed such plans, the level of concreteness of performance indicators and actual interventions varies substantially between the municipalities (e.g. Kommunernes Landsforening, 2014a). A recent survey shows that most municipalities have developed specific implementation plans for each of the 11 prevention packages issued by the Health Authority (N. Christiansen et al., 2015, p. 6). Moreover, almost all municipalities have established cross-sectoral collaboration within the municipalities to strengthen the implementation of the health prevention packages and other health promotion efforts. Yet the report also notes that many municipalities – in particular the smaller ones – still face problems developing coherent cross-sectoral health interventions.

Secondly, *key municipal welfare institutions should develop plans and initiatives encouraging more physical exercise and better diet*. Apart from such plans, kindergartens, schools, and nursing homes are also urged to pay attention to stigmatizing behaviour, i.e. the bullying of obese children and young persons. In order to make such initiatives successful, the management of these institutions must ensure that their staff receive the necessary education (Sundhedsstyrelsen, 2013, p. 19). In 2014, the level of physical activity for children at state schools was given a boost when the law governing state schools was changed as part of a wider school reform. Apart from the general extension of the school day, such schools must ensure that their pupils engage in at least 45 minutes of exercise each day (Law on Public Schools no. 665, 20 June 2014, §15). A year later, however, this regulation was still not fully implemented in many schools (Kommunernes Landsforening, 2015a).

Thirdly, the municipalities should conduct *early tracing of obesity among pre-school children* by municipal health services. The services, which are usually made up of a number of nurses and social and health assistants, should be mobilized to spot early signs of obesity development among pre-school children. This entails paying visits to parents' homes and talking with them about the importance of proper diet and physical exercise. Such initiatives have been developed in a number of municipalities (Høje-Taastrup Kommune, 2005; Faaborg-Midtfyn Kommune, 2013).

Fourthly, municipalities should develop *targeted and integrated programmes for obese or at-risk children, young people, and adults.* The first step is to spot the obese and those at risk. Municipal health nurses who pay regular visits to kindergartens and schools are therefore key individuals in identifying children and young people at risk. Adults are often identified by their general practitioner, who admits the person at risk to the municipality's course on how best to reduce weight in a sustainable manner (Sundhedsstyrelsen, 2013, p. 23). The second step is to develop and implement effective courses and programmes for these groups. In the case of obese children, such programmes should ideally include the parents, other close relatives, the health nurse, the school, and social authorities (Kommunernes Landsforening, 2015b, pp. 33–34). Thus, Local Government Denmark envisages a targeted programme spinning a dense network of relations between relevant actors that works in tandem to make the obese child (and her parents) change their lifestyle. Today, most if not all municipalities have developed such programmes, though their scope, design, and effectiveness vary immensely (Sundhedsstyrelsen, 2012e). Below, we examine two of these programmes in more depth.

Finally, municipalities should provide *easy access to information* about obesity control practices to both civil servants and to citizens. Today, all municipalities are using the new nationwide public digital citizen service (www.borger.dk) to provide quick overviews of the available and relevant health services in order to empower citizens to seek out the right service. Municipal employees are encouraged to access relevant information and share experiences using the nationwide digital health information services, including one about general health (www.sundhed.dk) and one about proper diet (www.altomkost.dk). As with many of the other municipal efforts in this area, there are a number of complaints and ongoing debates within the municipalities about how to improve ease of access to relevant information and services catering to particular health problems and target groups.

In brief, since the mid-2000s, Denmark has seen the development of a national action plan for controlling obesity. Following the structural reform of 2007, all Danish municipalities have stepped up their obesity-control interventions. In line with the general health promotion approach, these interventions have followed two distinct but highly interrelated prongs: interventions targeting obese individuals and interventions targeting the environment of the obese. As we shall see in more detail below, the former are characterized not only by biomedical advice on physical exercise and dieting but also by psychological expertise, which largely attributes obesity to a low level of self-esteem. The second prong is particularly interesting as it targets the environment not only of the obese but in principle of all citizens. Accordingly, the goal is not only to make the obese lose weight but also to prevent any (other) person from becoming obese. Here it is interesting to note that while there has been a lot of talk about the potential of nudging in the fight against obesity, this instrument has so far played a very limited role in the interventions launched by the Danish public health authorities.[2]

The biopolitical turn of the gymnastics movement

As mentioned above, the gymnastics movement was actively engaged in propagating physical exercise and bodily culture in Danish society from the early twentieth century. This movement, which also dealt with controlling obesity, was and still is entirely private, though it does receive some public support. Moreover, until the early 2000s, the strategies, programmes, and institutions propagated by gymnastics and sports organizations to promote physical exercise and bodily culture were not linked to the political strategies of the public health authorities.

In the early 2000s, the central management of the DGI decided to change its overall goal and strategy in order to enhance its own role in ensuring the promotion of good health among Danes. Over the next few years, the DGI central management would increasingly urge its local member associations to develop collaborative strategies and programmes in the area of health promotion and the prevention of lifestyle diseases (Vucina, 2014, pp. 173–174). This included fighting obesity. Collaboration with municipalities, schools, and workplaces was to be developed with a view towards providing adequate opportunities for physical exercise attuned to local needs. Above all, these opportunities were to be offered not only to the members of the gymnastics and sports associations but to every citizen in the local area.

One can speculate about the reason for the DGI's decision to link up with the public authorities' (state and municipalities) quest for health promotion and obesity control. Dwindling membership and fear of losing public financial support seem to be likely reasons. The structural reform of 2007, which charged municipalities with the task of ensuring health promotion, may have been regarded by the DGI as a window of opportunity to reinvigorate its role in local communities. Finally, we should not dismiss a genuine concern for the health of local citizens as a powerful motive driving the DGI decision as well. Whatever the reasons, the result was to bring the private non-profit sector wholesale into the political fight against obesity. In a coordinated effort with the municipalities, the key role for the DGI and its member associations was to reach as many local citizens as possible to engage them in a physically active lifestyle (Vucina, 2014, p. 174).

The strategic reorientation of the DGI subsequently resulted in the forging of a number of partnerships with various municipalities around the goal of undertaking a wide range of health promotion projects. The character, scope, and magnitude of these projects vary substantially. In the following discussion, we describe three schemes in order illustrate the diversity of DGI partnerships and interventions. The schemes also illustrate the two key sites of interventions in most contemporary health promotion programmes in Denmark: the interiority or subjectivity of individual citizens and the exteriority or the institutional environment supposedly shaping the choice of lifestyle.

Firstly, a health sports (*sundhedsidræts*) programme for people with back problems and cardiovascular diseases was established in 2015 in cooperation with five municipalities (DGI, 2016a). The programme targets physically inactive municipal residents deemed at risk of rheumatic and cardiovascular diseases. The programme interventions are conducted by specially trained coaches who focus not only on physiological dimensions of training but also the pedagogic and psychosocial dimensions that are deemed relevant to activate citizens with little motivation to exercise. This multidisciplinary approach is based on medical research on how best to motivate hitherto inactive citizens to take up and continue to engage in systematic physical activity. This programme illustrates that to the DGI health promotion is not only about making citizens engage in regular physical exercise, such as gymnastics or sports, but also about working on the mental dispositions of citizens in order to motivate and instil in them an attitude in which regular physical activity is a socially desirable norm of conduct.

Secondly, a set of programmes revolves around (voluntary) certification schemes targeting all Danish municipal day care institutions and schools. In order to become DGI certified, the institution will cooperate with the DGI to develop physical facilities and methods for play, movement, and various forms of sports with a view towards instilling a culture of physical exercise in the everyday life of the institution (DGI, 2016b, 2016c). The DGI stresses that physical exercise at kindergarten and in school contributes to the 'cognitive, motoric, social, mental and emotional development' of the child and instils in the child a propensity for life-long physical activity (DGI, 2016c).

Finally, the DGI offers to help municipalities and local voluntary organizations (mostly but not exclusively in the area of sports) to develop strategies for boosting their physical exercise activities (DGI, 2016d). The rationale of this programme is to develop and/or consolidate the relations between a wide range of local community actors – both public and private – to make it easier for local citizens to engage in some kind of regular physical activity. To meet this end, the programme assists local organizations in expanding their network, building and exchanging knowledge, mobilizing resources, increasing their visibility and communication, and ultimately strengthening their capacity to undertake long-term tasks in the area of supplying physical exercise facilities and programmes for local citizens. It is thus noteworthy that the DGI has expanded its scope from direct provision of physical exercise activities to also include organizational capacity-building and the forging of local networks of institutions that will make it easier and more obvious for citizens to engage in regular physical activity.

Case 1: Seize the Chance project

One of the outcomes of the DGI's decision to link up with the biopolitical fight against obesity was the Seize the Chance (*Grib chancen*) project targeting obese children and young people. The project involves a wide range of actors conducting the intervention and addresses the problem of obesity not only in physical and biomedical terms but also in psychological and social ones. The Seize the Chance project is above all targeting *the environment* of the obese.

The project was launched in 2009 by the Funen branch of the DGI in order to form a partnership with municipalities, sports clubs, the University of Southern Denmark, and other relevant actors in the region of Southern Denmark (Vucina, 2014, pp. 177–181). Its aim was to establish at least 30 interventions controlling child and youth obesity within a three-year period, by the end of which these interventions should be sustainable, i.e. continued and financed by the local municipalities or their partners. The project was divided into four phases (Idrætspolitisk Forum Fyn, 2010). Firstly, it generated knowledge, established contacts with interested municipalities, sports associations, schools, and after-school care institutions, and developed a model and forum for the partnership collaboration. It turned out that eight out of ten municipalities in the region decided to participate and provide financial support. Secondly, it launched dialogue meetings between the participating municipalities and sports associations. Thirdly, it consolidated the project design and secured the implementation structure of the various obesity-prevention interventions. Finally, the initiatives were anchored among the participating actors, and data were collected in order to allow the University of Southern Denmark to evaluate the project (Storm, Madsen, and Ibsen, 2012).

Apart from creating a more or less dense network of relevant actors and institutions involved in obesity control, the Seize the Chance project entailed that the participating schools and after-care institutions would help to spot obese children (all fifth-graders would go through a screening) and pass their names on to local sports associations. The municipalities would assist the sports associations in developing tailor-made physical activities for those kids that would enrol. The sports associations were not wholly convinced of the project strategy and refused to take orders from the municipal health service on how to deal with the obese children and youth. This conflict had largely been anticipated by the project steering committee, which urged municipalities to respect the sports associations and their particular approaches and to enter into a dialogue encouraging a mutual understanding about how best to deal with the kids. Based on its own premise, the project was not fully successful (Storm et al., 2012, pp. 29–32). While more than 30 interventions were launched, only few of these were anchored, in the sense of being continued and financed by the involved actors after the project terminated in 2012. Moreover, the number of kids participating in the activities offered by the sports associations was much lower than expected. The most significant durable effect seems to be the development of new contacts and consolidation of existing relationships between municipalities' health sections, schools, and sports associations.

In sum, at the most general level, the Seize the Chance project aimed to create a dense and durable network of public and private actors and institutions. These actors and institutions would, in turn, form a grid identifying the obese child or youth and offer her a set of physical activities and diet advice that would help her control her weight and regain self-esteem. The project was partially successful in doing that. Yet the project evaluation also showed that obese kids and their families are not as compliant with contemporary norms of health and vigour as desired by the biopolitical apparatus of state authorities, municipalities, schools, sports associations, and medical science.

Case 2: the Holbæk model

The so-called Holbæk model is another example of a coordinated intervention targeting obese children and young persons. This model has been widely acclaimed as a showcase for how to effectively tackle obesity. Thus, the example is not a typical but rather an extreme case of the fight against obesity. It is therefore useful not for generalizing but for illuminating how the power ingrained in health promotion may unfold when it is pushed to its limits.

In January 2008, the Unit for Obese Children and Young Persons was established at the paediatric section of Holbæk Hospital (Henningsen and Dyhrberg, 2009). In cooperation with the Holbæk municipality, an interdisciplinary team of paediatricians, genetic specialists, nurses, clinical dietitians, psychologists, and social counsellors worked together to diagnose, counsel, and treat obese children and young persons. Apart from this interdisciplinary tack, the Holbæk model implied active involvement of the parents of the obese children. The goal of the interdisciplinary team is to ensure that all persons treated stabilized their weight and gradually approached a normal-range BMI. Moreover, they explicitly reject what they saw as the prevalent defeatist attitude among many of their colleagues, who found that many obese people cannot not be helped because they lack the interest or will to do something about their condition. By the end of 2014 the paediatric department at Holbæk Hospital had treated more than 1,900 children and young persons, of whom around 80 per cent had lost weight for a longer period (Den Korte Avis, 2014). Accordingly, by early 2016, at least 14 municipalities had adopted the model (Region Sjælland, 2014; Egedal Kommune, 2015; Sønderborg Nyt, 2015; Syddjurs Kommune, 2015; Odder Kommune, 2016).[3] Moreover, similar integrated techniques targeting the whole family in order to create sustainable weight losses with obese children have been developed in other municipalities, such as Copenhagen (Kommunernes Landsforening, 2014b).

The intervention entailed by the Holbæk model has three core characteristics that are seen as vital to its success: integrative, long-term, and positive. Firstly and above all, the Holbæk model is a technique integrating several aspects of everyday conduct of the obese. It is considered inadequate to look only at the child's diet or habits of physical activity. The nurse and social counsellor will also look into the social and peer relations of the obese child, her self-esteem, her performance in school, etc. In particular, the obese child's parents are given advice on how to make healthy meals and encourage their child to engage in physical exercise (Strøm, 2012). Thus, obesity is not considered to be only a physical or medical problem but also a psychological and social one. This is why the psychologist and social counsellor will engage in dialogue with the obese child, his parents, schoolteachers, and perhaps even peers. Secondly, the intervention has to be long-term, involving regular visits by the staff every two months or so for at least one year to monitor progress and adjust the interventions. Finally, inspired by positive psychology, all the staff meet both the obese child and her parents not with negative attitudes and judgments but with a positive attitude looking for successes and positive feelings that may encourage durable changes in the child's lifestyle. Again, this includes making the parents adopt a positive approach towards their child and focus on rewards rather than on negative sanctions.

Interestingly, the Holbæk model is based not only on psychosocial conceptions of obesity but also hereditary or, more precisely, genetic ones. Thus, a biobank containing genetic profiles both of the obese treated in the municipality of Holbæk and a control group (of non-obese) has been developed to unravel the complex interactions between social and genetic factors behind the development of obesity (Holm, 2016). On the one hand, participation in genetic screening is voluntary.

On the other hand, the fact that almost all children going through the treatment process provide a sample for genetic screening indicates that their parents are subjected to some fairly strong arguments from medical personnel. So far, it has been noted that differences in individual setup may influence hormone balances and perhaps even gastric bacterial cultures, which in turn influence metabolism and, ultimately, weight (Holm, 2015). However, apart from experiments with modifying gastric bacterial cultures, genetic screening has not really impacted the predominantly psychosocial therapeutic approach described above.

In sum, the Holbæk model constitutes a mode of intervention that directly and explicitly trespasses on the liberally invented private sphere of the family to bring about durable changes of conduct. Moreover, it works not only by providing biomedical expert advice but also – and perhaps more importantly – by working on the attitude and routines making up the everyday life of the obese child and his family, i.e. by making them freely subject themselves to the norms of a healthy lifestyle. Accordingly, even if almost all children treated at the paediatric clinic at Holbæk Hospital are subjected to genetic screening to unravel the interaction between social and biological factors behind their obesity, there is so far no indication that this has any significant impact on the preferred treatment methods, namely various forms psychosocial counselling working through the self-esteem of the obese child and her parents.

Conclusion

This chapter has examined the fight against obesity in Denmark. We have shown that this fight is part and parcel of the wider turn towards health promotion that emerged as a generalized strategy during the 1990s. Accordingly, the key governing techniques targeting the obese have not been legally sanctioned bans or dictates. Rather, on the one hand, we have seen the rise of psychological techniques seeking to control obesity by increasing the self-esteem of the obese combined with practical advice on how to make physical exercise and healthy eating a part of the everyday routines of the obese individual and her family. On the other hand, we have seen the development of collaborative networks between municipalities and a range of other public and private actors. The rationale here is to develop an institutional grid of actors and initiatives that will make a healthy lifestyle the obvious choice of every Danish citizen, not just those already obese.

As with many of the other health promotion strategies, we should be wary of exaggerating the efficacy of the fight against obesity. Both national surveys and experiences from individual projects, such as the two cases explored above, show that these programmes fail over and over again to meet their own ambitions. Accordingly, until recently, the number of overweight and obese Danes has kept growing. Yet we still think there is a need for concern here, because we find a widespread political agreement over the desirability of building a tight-knit and durable network encouraging each child and young person in Danish society to choose a healthy lifestyle. The predominant political support for this totalizing mode of health promotion is sustained by contemporary medical science both inside Denmark and outside (the WHO). Accordingly, when the fight against obesity fails to reach its objectives, this has been taken by Danish health authorities, municipalities, and various private organizations not as a reason to drop the strategy or even to revise it. Instead, these failures are taken as an indication of the need to develop and consolidate the health promotion strategy even further. In fact, the most important critique of the fight against obesity seems to come neither from politicians nor from (medical and social) scientists, but from the many obese children – and their parents – who refuse to actively participate in the schemes that are supposed to do them good.

How can we understand this persistence of health promotion strategies in face of their many failures and economic expenditures? High public expenditure with little or no positive societal economic impact, such as agricultural subsidies, are often explained by political scientists in terms of vested interests and the asymmetry between concentrated benefits (e.g. to farmers) and dispersed costs (imposed on taxpayers) (cf. Wilson, 1980, pp. 367–370). However, in the case of health promotion, both the costs and benefits are long-term and dispersed. Accordingly, we do not find well-organized private interest groups fighting for more public money to support health promotion interventions. Thus, the explanation does not seem to lie in interest-group politics.

There must then be some other political force or rationale at play inducing politicians to invest heavily in costly health interventions, the effects of which have not been systematically documented. Our suggestion is that the contemporary quest for health promotion and obesity control is informed by a wider political rationality of activism and empowerment. This rationality, which is also found in areas of education and unemployment regulation (Dean, 1995; Triantafillou, 2012), essentially regards societal problems like obesity as a question of inactive and disempowered citizens. This political rationality has been dubbed 'constructivist neoliberalism', a term denoting the kind of rationality that regards the role of the state to be an enabling and empowering one, working to stimulate the self-steering capacities of individuals, groups, and organizations (Triantafillou, 2017). According to this rationality, people are fat because they are inactive, and people are inactive because they are disempowered. The latter entails not only insufficient economic resources and little education but also substance abuse problems, few and fragile social relations, and above all low self-esteem. If the problem is inactivity and disempowerment, then the solution is always some kind of intervention seeking to activate and empower the obese.

This constructivist neoliberal rationality in itself cannot explain the fight against obesity by way of health promotion. In order to understand this fight, it is important to note the way in which obesity was singled out as a biopolitical problem through epidemiological studies from the 1990s onwards. The studies provided the clear message that the health and vigour of the Danish population was under threat from the growing percentage of obese people. In particular, the growing medical knowledge linking obesity to diabetes, cardiovascular diseases, and certain forms of cancer made it difficult for politicians not to react. Moreover, unlike in the 1920s and 1930s, obesity was not inscribed in racial discourses of heritage and biological predispositions. Instead, physiological knowledge was overlapped by pedagogic and psychological discourses seeing obesity as a sign not of racial degeneration but of a combination of inadequate education, poor social relations, and low self-esteem. The strategic linking of these scientific discourses with the wider neoliberal rationalities contributed to making health promotion the obvious political strategy in the fight against obesity.

In rapport with this constructivist neoliberalism, it seems to us that a certain form of optimistic vitalism is at play in the Danish fight against obesity. This is a frugal vitalism in the sense that is eschews excessive body weight, excessive eating, and a general lack of self-control. Yet it is also an optimistic vitalism in the sense that it assumes that all Danes, not only the overweight and the obese, can constantly improve their health and vigour by improving their diet, their physical exercise, their self-esteem, and their engagement with family, peers, colleagues, and civil society organizations. It is also optimistic in the sense that even though a fairly coherent and well-financed public health apparatus has been established (at least when compared to the English case examined in the previous chapter), Danish public health authorities, medical experts, and numerous civil society organizations argue that it is both possible and desirable to further improve the health and vigour of Danes by further reforming and streamlining interventions tailored to the individual and her needs.

Notes

1 The analysis of the fight against obesity is based on a more or less systematic compilation of policy and expert documents located by going through the homepages of the Ministry of Health, the Danish National Health Authority, the State Institute of Public Health, the National Association of Municipalities, and the Danish Institute for Local and Regional Government Research. We

have not made systematic reviews of biomedical journals as our main interest is in the concrete political rationalities and techniques seeking to prevent obesity, rather than the strictly medical-curative techniques, such as liposuction and gastric bypass.
2 We managed to find only one concrete nudging-based intervention in the area of obesity control in the municipality of Langeland (Kommunernes Landsforening, 2014c).
3 The following municipalities have adopted the Holbæk model: Egedal, Faurskov, Hedensted, Holbæk, Horsens, Kalundborg, Kolding, Norddjurs, Odder, Randers, Slagelse, Sønderborg, Stevns, Syddjurs, and Vejle.

5
Promoting recovery in England

This chapter examines the political rationalities, expertise, and techniques of government involved in the emergence of mental recovery in England as a field of more or – very often – less systematic political intervention. As in many other liberal democracies, the treatment of the mentally ill in England has undergone a substantial transformation from an approach in which relatively narrow biomedical interventions were employed in large-scale mental institutions to so-called community-based care. This implies comprehensive interventions focusing not only on the clinical status of the mentally ill but also on their family, social, and housing situations (Department of Health, 1999, p. 47). These complex interventions are orchestrated by community health teams with a view towards assisting the patient in living a life that is as full as possible (Department of Health, 2001, p. 4). Within this wider transition, recovery has increasingly been offered as means for assisting the mentally ill with living a better, if not symptom-free, life outside the great institutions (Roberts et al., 2006b, p. xvi). The recovery approach is by definition a comprehensive operation that relies on multi-agency and multi-disciplinary interventions, community-based work (Wing and Morris, 1981, p. 148; WHO, 2001, pp. 110–111), and cross-sectorial collaboration (Mountain and Holloway, 2007, p. 4, Kalidindi, Killaspy, and Edwards, 2012, p. 12).

Our overall argument in this chapter is that recovery is a power-laden practice that works above all through nurturing and structuring the self-steering capacities – the freedom – of the mentally ill. While we strongly sympathize with those that celebrate the emancipatory potential of the de-institutionalization of the treatment of mental illness, we are also concerned with the new kind of power ingrained in the recovery approach. Firstly, the mentally ill are now expected to constantly work on their self in order to live a fuller life. Many recovery proponents stress that the goal of this self-reflection is not to become normal or cured – in the sense of being free from symptoms. Instead, they argue that the patient should pursue her dreams and happiness. Nevertheless, even these rather radical proponents of recovery insist that the patient should constantly reflect on how she can improve the ways in which she lives with her disease. The logical implication is that this self-steering or ethical practice should only stop once the patient is no longer ill, or when she is able to nurture family relations, take care of her housing situation, and attend a regular, paid job.

Secondly, the inter-organizational and interdisciplinary approach that makes up recovery rests on a regulatory ideal in which the community or the social fabric at large is saturated by a dense web of governmental institutions and relations that constantly work to empower and thereby to recover the mentally ill. Thus, while the mentally ill have been emancipated from what Erving Goffman termed the 'total institutions' (Goffman, 1961), they are now enmeshed in a more or less dense web of governmental institutions and relations that strive to cover every aspect of the life of the mentally ill. When these institutions fail to address the conduct of the mentally ill, which the many tragic stories of suicide and violence testify to, then this is taken as an argument for further improving in the sense of tightening the seams of the recovery apparatus.

The chapter unfolds in the following way: after a brief account of the historical antecedents of contemporary recovery, we analyse the psychosocial turn of the treatment of mental illness in England. This involves mapping key political rationalities and the new way of conceiving mental illness through an expanding range of expertise. We then move on to account for some of the actual programmes and techniques employed in recovery treatment. Finally, we sum up and discuss our findings.

Historical antecedents

During the first half of the nineteenth century, the Quaker philanthropist and mental health reformer William Tuke was in charge of the York Retreat for insane persons, commonly referred to as the Retreat. The Retreat opened in 1796 (Tuke, 1813, p. 45) and came to be an exemplary case of a method that Tuke's grandson Samuel Tuke later termed 'moral treatment'. At the centre of attention was the patient's ability to recover from her insanity and ensuring the general wellbeing of the patients (Tuke, 1813, pp. 138). Moral treatment hinged on the self-steering powers of the patients. An essential part of this treatment was to show kindness and trust in the patient (Tuke, 1813, p. 136):

> We have already observed that the most insane persons have a considerable degree of self command; and that the employment and elevation

of this remaining power found to be attached with the most salutary effects. (Tuke, 1813, pp. 139–140)

Tuke's moral treatment indicates that recovery understood as an enhancement of the capacity of the mentally ill person to govern herself and her disease through therapeutic intervention is not an entirely new phenomenon. While Tuke's moral treatment was never very successful, it became a very significant idea in the critical debate over the use of coercive methods in the treatment of the mentally ill (Shorter, 1997, p. 21). There are probably few if any direct links between Tuke's moral treatment two centuries ago and contemporary recovery, though one of the central promoters of recovery in England, the Royal College of Psychiatrists in London, claims to be inspired by William Tuke (Roberts and Wolfson, 2006, p. 19).

A more contemporary source of inspiration for recovery, though no less ambiguous than Tuke's moral treatment, is psychoanalysis. While psychoanalysis originated as a therapy with strictly biomedical aspirations that aimed to cure the patient of neurotic and psychotic disorders, it came increasingly to foster ideas of self-determination. By insisting on the active role of the patient in her care of going through traumas and inducing transference, psychoanalysis has always relied on the patient being an active participant rather than a passive object of treatment. Of course, there are tremendous differences between various strands of twentieth-century psychoanalysis regarding the role attributed to the patient, but many insist that the patient must actively take part in her own care. Even if it is granted that psychoanalytic treatments hinge more or less directly on the recuperation of the patient's self-government, one may object that psychoanalysis had rather limited resonance in the treatment of mental illness in England (Rayner, 1990). Also, the number of practising psychoanalysts and psychotherapists in Britain may be no more than 1,500 (British Psychoanalytic Council, 2017).

While psychoanalysis may never have pervaded the treatment of mental illness in Britain as effectively as in the US or in France, it has not been unimportant either. Psychoanalytic treatment was formally accepted and entitled to financial support from the NHS as early as 1948 (O. Olsen and Køppe, 1996, p. 424). This support has sustained, for example, the still-active Portman Clinic, which was opened in London in 1933 by the Institute for the Study and Treatment of Delinquency to treat delinquent and criminal patients. It is still operating and still using psychoanalytic therapy – since 1994 in concert with the Tavistock Institute (Valiér, 1998). British psychoanalysis is renowned for its development of new approaches to children's mental diseases during the interwar period by Melanie Klein and Anna Freud. It also played a key role in the work on group theory advanced by Wilfred Bion through the Tavistock Institute both prior to and following World War II (N. Rose, 1989). Moreover, paediatrician and psychoanalyst Donald Winnicott popularized the importance of maternal care for the child's psychological development through pamphlets, public lectures, and radio broadcasts during the 1940s and 1950s (cf. Schwartz, 1999, p. 242).

Ironically, the most significant thrust for integrating the patient's subjective experiences and active engagement into the curative process seems to have come not from the trained psychoanalysts but from the Scottish psychiatrist Ronald D. Laing. Inspired by Gregory Bateson, Laing would understand schizophrenia as a transitory journey during which the patient would try to communicate his distress and worries by what to others appeared to be completely incomprehensible modes of communication (Laing, 1960). Accordingly, therapy should entail that maximum efforts be made to understand the concerns expressed by the patient, seen from the point of view of the patient's concrete experiences. The follow-up after the – often tentative – cure almost reads as a contemporary recovery approach textbook:

> Preparation for the person's return to his family and community requires work with his family and other social networks before he leaves hospital, as well as thereafter. Continuity of care is required, without the existing tendency to separate, economically and organizationally, the 'cure' of the 'illness' from the 'care of the person'. (Laing, 1964, p. 192)

Of course, Laing's ideas of treatment of the severely mentally ill were slow to permeate into state-sanctioned treatment practice. Both the empowerment of the patient and the mobilization of the community in that process would be some three decades away.

The Mental Health Act of 1959 marked one of the first tiny signals of change in government policy from a relatively narrow biomedical focus to a more interdisciplinary approach that provided care outside the hospital setting (Department of Health, 2001, p. 4). Then, during the 1970s, a number of day hospitals and decentralized acute wards were established as an alternative to institutionalization. The 1980s saw the launching of community mental health teams, often initiated by private bodies such as MIND and the National Schizophrenic Fellowship. While these attempts often had little to do with traditional psychoanalysis, they shared the notion that the care for the mentally ill was not solely to be left to psychiatrists and that the patient was to take a much more active role in his cure than had hitherto been the case in the prevailing biomedical therapies.

In brief, while trained British psychoanalysts may have played a rather limited role in espousing the rationales underlying recovery, the psychoanalytical approach of paying attention to the patient's subjective experience and active participation in her cure both inside and, increasingly, outside clinical and hospital settings was pushed by British psychiatrists, psychotherapists, and other reformers from the 1960s.

Empowering the patient

Since the 1990s, a number of medical practitioners and others involved in mental health care have written on recovery. In this vast literature, we often encounter a distinction between 'recovery' and 'rehabilitation'. Recovery is usually defined as an approach by which people suffering from mental illness are offered various empowerment techniques in order to better cope with their illness and be able to lead a better life (Anthony and Farkas, 1982; Anthony, 1993, 2004; Harrison et al., 2001, p. 517; A. Kelly and Gamble, 2005, pp. 247–248). Rehabilitation, in turn, is often defined as the means (programmes, procedures, and techniques) by which recovery is to take place. While these means range from antipsychotic medical treatment to community services, their key rationale is to create and sustain a psychosocial support system outside the clinical setting (WHO, 2001, pp. xi–xiii, 62). Or, as Pat Deegan asserts in 1988: 'rehabilitation is a professional and service process while recovery is the desired outcome' (see Roberts et al., 2006b, p. xv). In the following, unless a point is made to separate the two, we use the term recovery to cover both the aspiration to empower the mentally ill and the diverse range of programmes, procedures, and techniques informed by this aspiration.

In line with the international trends of recovery, we see a recovery approach reflected in the clinical guidelines for English mental health promoted by the National Institute for Clinical Excellence, later named National Institute for Health and Care Excellence (NICE). NICE produces standardized recommendations for clinical practice for public health and social care services in the UK, recommendations that are adopted also by other countries, the Danish Health Authority and the Danish psychiatric services included (http://sundhedsstyrelsen.dk/da/soeg?q=nice; www.regioner.dk/soeg?q=nice). In the NICE guidelines from 2002, a whole chapter is dedicated to the promotion of recovery. NICE argues that, with treatment, the majority of people tend to improve or recover (National Institute for Clinical Excellence, 2002, p. 36). The instruments of recovery include assertive outreach teams for people with serious mental disorder, including people with schizophrenia. They cover a range of psychological and psychosocial interventions from cognitive behavioural therapy and family intervention for relapse prevention and symptom reduction to antipsychotic drugs and the search for employment opportunities (National Institute for Clinical Excellence, 2002, pp. 13–21; Drake and Whitley, 2014, p. 242).

Mike Slade, an influential advocate for recovery, has published a guide for recovery intervention in community-based mental health teams in England that is also used in Denmark. Slade emphasizes recovery as a 'person-centred' process (Slade, 2013, p. 4) by which a psychosocial approach must be adapted to individual needs. Slade argues that in recovery there is 'no ideal or "right" service' (Slade, 2013, p. 5) but a variety of possible means and outcomes. This approach follows the assumption that the mentally ill individual is capable of managing his own life (Slade, 2013, p. 13). As Slade asserts: 'You can do it – we can help' (Slade, 2013, pp. 17, 26). This kind of empowerment entails that the so-called service user is the decision-maker (Slade, 2013, p. 13) who is engaged in a process towards personal responsibility (Slade, 2013, p. 20) and self-management (Slade, 2013, p. 25) within a respectful and welcoming environment (Slade, 2013, p. 25). Here, the carer is less an expert and more a coach. Accordingly, recovery-orientated service is a matter of coaching or facilitating the process of recovery and enabling the amplification of strength rather than deficits (Slade, 2013, p. 13) as well as developing and validating personal meaning for the service user (Slade, 2013, p. 18). The professional–service relationship is then a kind of partnership (Slade, 2013, p. 20). This twofold approach of addressing both individual competences and environmental change is generally found (Wing and Morris, 1981, p. 133; National Collaboration Centre for Mental Health, 2014, p. 28) – which we elaborate in the subsequent section – and is also in tune with the WHO's recommendations. As stated by the WHO: 'The main objectives are consumers' empowerment and reduction of discrimination and stigma, the improvement of social competences' (WHO, 2001, p. 62). It is emphasized that recovery is in fact an individual experience of personal growth and change and an attitude to approaching daily life (A. Kelly and Gamble, 2005, p. 246), emphasizing the importance of everyday activities, routines, and life processes (Drake and Whitley, 2014, p. 236).

Secondly, as emphasized by Mike Slade, recovery as a person-centred process entails an explicit use of mentally disabled individuals as experts in their disease. The recovery process in this way takes its point of departure in personal experiences of mentally ill people (Slade, 2013, p. 6). Personal recovery thus alludes to drawing from people with 'lived experience' of mental illness (Slade, 2013, p. 8). The patients then are 'experts by experience' (Crane, 2003, quoted in Roberts and Wolfson, 2006, p. 19). Experience is regarded as an essential point of departure for the recovery process. This approach to recovery has implications for the mental health profession. Thus, Roberts and Wolfson refer to a recent selection for president of the Royal College of Psychiatrists, by which a recent president in seeking re-election included his personal experience of depression (Roberts and Wolfson, 2006, p. 19). Using service users' expertise is taken to the level where a psychiatric department includes people in recovery from mental illness as educators (Bender, 2012, p. 14). Also, the WHO promotes peer support as an important means of recovery (WHO, 2001, p. 56).

The term used in England is *peer specialist* or *peer support*, sometimes referred to as 'survivor accounts' (A. Kelly and Gamble, 2005, p. 248): that is, someone who has succeeded in recovering from mental illness and functions as a peer for those in process of recovery (Bender, 2012, p. 15). Peer support has been a part of English mental health services since around 2000 (Olesen, 2015, p. 21). That year, the Department of Health launched *The Expert Patient* as a new approach to chronic disease management in the twenty-first century (Department of Health, 2000, p. 6; Department of Health, 2001). The announcement reads:

> [R]esearch and practical experience in North America and Britain are showing that today's patients with chronic disease need not be mere recipients of care. They can become a decision-maker in the treatment process. (Department of Health, 2000, p. 5)

This elevation of the patient as an expert in her own illness is contrasted with a traditional clinical approach. While a clinician can establish a diagnosis, the patient has the experience of illness; the clinician looks for disease aetiology, while a patient-centred approach is concerned with social circumstance. Moreover, whereas the clinical approach operates with prognosis in the sense of more or less objective calculations of the probability of cure, the patient-centred approach operates with the patient's subjective attitude to risk. Finally, while a clinician speaks of outcome in the sense of the degree to which symptoms are reduced, the patient-centred approach emphasizes values and life quality (Department of Health, 2000, p. 11). This opposition between the clinical and the recovery approach finds support among various recovery advocates (Roberts and Wolfson, 2006, p. 20). Mike Slade has formulated the distinction between the two approaches in the following way: clinical recovery emerges from the expertise of mental health professionals and involves getting rid of symptoms, restoring social functioning, and getting back to normal (Slade, 2013, p. 8). In contrast, personal recovery emerges from the expertise of people with lived experience and is therefore a personal, unique process of changing one's attitudes, values, feelings, goals, skills, and roles (Slade, 2013, 10).

By implication, the new recovery approach hinges on the activation or the empowerment of the patient in her own healing process. This is not to say that biomedical expertise and professionals, such as psychiatrists, are superfluous. However, their key role is no longer (only) to provide objective diagnosis and therapies that essentially deal with the patient as an object (a thing). Rather, the medical profession has to engage the patient and mobilize her experience, knowledge, and resources in an attempt to reduce symptoms and, above all, enable the patient to handle symptoms that it may not be possible to cure, in a way that allows her to live a richer and fuller life.

Recovery ad infinitum? Empowering the schizophrenic patient

It would seem obvious to assume that recovery is applied only to the milder forms of mental illness and that more severe illnesses are left to traditional biomedical approaches. At least, that was our initial assumption. However, this is not the case. In fact, schizophrenia, which may be one of the most disturbing and difficult – if not outright impossible – to cure mental illnesses has increasingly become the object of recovery approaches. We take this as an indication of just how strong the recovery approach has positioned itself in the armoury of contemporary public health politics.

Since the Swiss psychiatrist Eugen Bleuler named schizophrenia in the early twentieth century, it has been widely assumed that the disease is chronic and that cure is rare (National Collaborating Centre for Mental Health, 2014, p. 17). In fact, some clinicians would argue that a cured case of schizophrenia is a contradiction in terms, and therefore the diagnosis must have been inaccurate in the first place (cf. Harding, Brooks, Ashikaka, Strauss, and Breier, 1987, p. 727). The difficulty of curing schizophrenia has been attributed partly to the severe, psychotic nature of the symptoms and partly to its hereditary nature. Even today schizophrenia is a somewhat blurry category and it is difficult to pinpoint symptoms accurately. That said, psychosis is a central symptom associated with the disease. However, psychosis does not equal schizophrenia, as other symptoms have to be present, too. Schizophrenia is often regarded as an attack on or an alteration of the individual's personality, mostly through states of hallucinations, distorted and bizarre ideas and speech, as well as behavioural disturbances (National Collaborating Centre for Mental Health, 2014, p. 14).

The notion of the incurable nature of schizophrenia has been increasingly questioned, which is reflected in the various versions of the two diagnostic systems used by health professionals in the Western world: the international classification of mental illness model ICD, published by the WHO, and the American diagnostic model Diagnostic and Statistical Manual of Mental Disorders (DSM). From the first editions of both ICD and DSM from the 1950s up until the latest revision – the latest ICD, ICD-10, was published in 1992, while the latest DSM, DSM-5, was published in 2013 – the chronic nature of schizophrenia has gradually been questioned. The acknowledgement of the possibility of a partial cure for at least some schizophrenic patients is linked to a shift in the understanding of its hereditary character. From its inception schizophrenia was seen as hereditary. However, with the genetic revolution, the understanding of heritage shifted from a largely deterministic one to a more probabilistic one where a certain genetic predisposition may be triggered by a wide range of epi-genetic or social factors, such as family relations, lifestyle, traumatic events, etc. (National Collaboration Centre for Mental Health, 2014, pp. 20–21).

The changing understanding of schizophrenia and its possible cure can be linked to a number of trials conducted between the 1960s and the 1980s, particularly in the US In 1965, Bleuer studied 208 individuals with schizophrenia and to his surprise found that 66 per cent recovered either partly or fully from their illness. Likewise, Ciompi and Huber in 1980 found that more than half of the patients diagnosed with schizophrenia recovered (see A. Kelly and Gamble, 2005, p. 247). More importantly, the findings of the 'Vermont longitudinal study' from 1987 seriously questioned the understanding of schizophrenia as a chronic mental illness (Harrison et al., 2001; Roberts and Wolfson, 2006; Kalidindi et al., 2012). The trial was the first of its kind in terms of the time frame and number of individuals subjected to the trial. A long-term follow-up study was made of 118 patients from Vermont State Hospital in the US, all admitted to hospital in the 1950s with the DSM diagnosis of schizophrenia (Harding et al., 1987, pp. 727–728). The study showed that between one third and two-thirds of the cohort had significantly improved or recovered. In fact, the follow-up study found that 68 per cent did not display any signs of symptoms of schizophrenia when assessed according to the DSM-3 criteria (Harding et al., 1987, p. 730). The Vermont study paved the way for a more optimistic view of the possibility of curing schizophrenia or at least reducing the severity of the symptoms. Yet it would take another decade before this more optimistic view of schizophrenia would coalesce with the new curative approach, recovery. This approach would break with the exclusive focus on removing symptoms and instead seek to augment the competences of the patient to handle her symptoms in a way that allowed her to live a more full life.

During the 2000s, both the WHO and the National Collaboration Centre for Mental Health began viewing schizophrenia and its treatment from a recovery perspective. In the *World Health Report. Mental Health: New Understanding, New Hope*, the WHO described how schizophrenia follows a much more variable course than previously assumed (WHO, 2001). According to the WHO, about one third of schizophrenia cases end with complete symptomatic and social cure. The rest follow a chronic or recurrent trajectory, which may lead to complete social recovery but are dependent on drug therapy and psychosocial care (WHO, 2001, p. 33), including housing, employment, and social support networks (WHO, 2001, p. 62). While the WHO and the National Collaboration Centre maintained that schizophrenia could not be prevented from emerging, they found it possible and desirable to arrest further advances of the disease (secondary prevention). Above all, they recommended that psychosocial care be provided to enable the patient to live a fuller life with his diseases (WHO, 2001, p. 68; National Collaborating Centre for Mental Health, 2014, p. 17).

This way of addressing schizophrenia, in terms of empowering the patient to cope with her symptoms, rather than trying – often in vain – to eliminate all symptoms, has had strong resonance in England. For example, the Department of Health suggests that the increased rate of recovery for individuals with schizophrenia should be seen in light of more effective medication available since the 1960s (Department of Health, 2001, p. 4). More recently, the National Collaborating Centre for Mental Health has identified recovery to increase the quality of life that is a potentiality related to even the most serious mental diseases like schizophrenia – 'recovery may happen any time, even after many years' (National Collaborating Centre for Mental Health, 2014, p. 18). Recovery is regarded less as a clinical system and more a psychosocial support system: 'emphasis has been on developing services that support people in achieving their own self-defined recovery goals' (National Collaborating Centre for Mental Health, 2014, p. 35). The recovery approach has been adopted by NICE, whose guidelines convey the message that everyone with a mental disability can potentially benefit from recovery (National Collaborating Centre for Mental Health, 2014, p. 101).

In short, a number of clinical findings from the 1960s onwards to the 1980s paved the way for a break with the chronic notion of schizophrenia. This loosening up of the clinical attitude towards schizophrenic patients correlated well with a recovery approach to mental illness; that is, if schizophrenia is not curable, then it is at least something one might recover from, in the broad sense of the term. The means emphasized then are less clinical measures than extra-clinical factors, such as a strong local community and social support as well as psychological techniques for strengthening the patient's self-esteem and ability to master her own life.

The psychosocial turn or invoking the community

Medical experts and public health authorities invariably link recovery to self-management and empowerment (Department of Health, 2000, p. 5; Roberts and Wolfson, 2006, p. 29; Drake and Whitley, 2014, p. 236). The role of professionals is to create an environment in which mental illness is managed through a number of coping strategies, i.e. mental illness self-management (National Collaborating Centre for Mental Health, 2014, p. 190). It is this link between recovery and extra-clinical interventions that we examine in the following section.

Somewhat paradoxically, the call for dealing with even severe forms of mental illness outside the clinical setting has come from within medicine or psychiatry itself. As mentioned above, recovery is perceived as a broad, multifaceted attitude towards mental illness in which psychosocial forms of knowledge and techniques are the centre of attention. In contrast, the biological model is depicted as an outdated medical attitude where clinical symptoms are the centre of attention. While this self-identification may help to boost the confidence and image of recovery, it does little to understand the developments in biomedicine. As it turns out, it is within medicine itself that we find some of the most outspoken supporters of recovery, arguing for a break with the 'medical model'. Many psychiatrists are now warning against the dangers of a narrow biological understanding and treatment of mental illness and for the need for broader approaches (A. Kelly and Gamble, 2005, p. 246).

As early as 1980, the Royal College of Psychiatrists published a document on psychiatric rehabilitation that argued for the need for a recovery approach (Wing and Morris, 1981, pp. 1, 147). The Faculty of Rehabilitation and Social Psychiatry, working under the Royal College of Psychiatrists, was established in 1997 in order to provide expert knowledge in the fields of rehabilitation and longer-term mental health conditions to the College, the Department of Health, service providers, and voluntary organizations (Roberts and Wolfson, 2006, pp. 33–34). Since then, the Faculty of Rehabilitation and Social Psychiatry, which consists of consultant psychiatrists, specialist doctors, trainee psychiatrists, service users, and care group representatives, has issued a number of strategy and evaluation documents calling for the improvement of rehabilitation and recovery services. The Faculty has often lamented what they see as poorly coordinated residential care and hospital services (Holloway, 2005, p. 1) and the absence of systematic strategies for recovery, rehabilitation, and long-term care interventions in the UK (Mountain and Holloway, 2007, p. 3).

This medical call for a broader approach to mental illness, including both biological and psychosocial dimensions, came more or less in tandem with New Labour community empowerment strategy from the late 1990s (N. Rose, 1999, pp. 192–193; Taylor, 2007). During the 2000s, local communities and governments were increasingly included as key actors in securing mental recovery in England. Mental health services in this period emphasized early intervention for young people in their first episode of psychosis, referred to as Early Intervention in Psychosis and Association Outreach Teams, as an example of a recovery approach

(Power, Smith, Shiers, and Roberts, 2006, p. 127). There has also been increased focus on family members, care professionals, and the community in the work conducted by the Department of Health and the National Service Framework for Mental Health (Department of Health, 1999). This framework set standards in four areas: health promotion, primary care, access to services for people with severe mental illness, and the prevention of suicide. This entailed the launching of so-called community psychosis services, including community rehabilitation teams and assertive outreach teams, which are another case of recovery at work (Kalidindi et al., 2012, p. 9). A progress report in 2007 by the Department of Health showed improvements in a number of mental health services, including a significant increase in the number of mental health staff and the provision of 700 new community mental health teams (Appleby, 2007). These are part of the nationwide community mental health teams (CMHT), a service directed at people with enduring psychosis (Kalidindi et al., 2012, p. 5). Northern England's regional version of CMHT has adopted recovery-orientated elements, inspired by a Dutch recovery model, which focus on more intensive, patient-centred care (Kalidindi et al., 2012, p. 6).

This emphasis on the role of the community in providing mental health services, developed under the New Labour government, was essentially continued by the Coalition government. For example, the Secretary of State's 2010 strategy for health recovery and rehabilitation plan stated:

> Centralisation has failed ... We will end this top-down government. It is time to free up local government and local communities to decide how best to improve the health and wellbeing of their citizens. (Secretary of State for Health, 2010, p. 25)

On the basis of this diagnosis, the Secretary of State announced that the new Coalition government would shift 'power to local communities enabling them to improve health throughout people's lives, reduce inequalities and focus on the needs of the local population' (Secretary of State for Health, 2010, p. 31). In line with this wider strategy of invoking the capacity of the local community, local rehabilitation inpatient beds and Community Rehabilitation Teams were increased all over England. Most National Health Teams consist of at least one community-based rehabilitation unit per local authority area, and over half of the NHS Trusts have a community-based rehabilitation team. Put differently, 25 per cent of the total mental health budget is absorbed by rehabilitation services for people with longer-term and complex mental health needs (Join Commissioning Panel for Mental Health, 2012, p. 11).

The emphasis on a patient-centred recovery approach and community mobilization has now permeated the official clinical guidelines. The National Collaborating Centre for Mental Health, which was established in the late 1990s by the NHS and the National Institute for Health and Care Excellence, endorses psychosocial interventions in order to promote recovery. These interventions should tap into a number of extra-clinical factors related to lifestyle and other factors in the local community (National Collaborating Centre for Mental Health, 2014, p. 32). Accordingly, the role of professionals is to create an environment in which mental illness is governed through a number of coping strategies, i.e. mental illness self-management (National Collaborating Centre for Mental Health, 2014, p. 190). Similarly, the mental health guidelines of the National Institute for Health and Care Excellence emphasize that the so-called 'support networks' of a patient be identified as one of the first steps in her treatment. Moreover, if a patient is transferred from a hospital to a community service, it is fundamental upon discharge to enable the person to maintain links with their home community (National Institute for Health and Care Excellence, 2016). This should be done by supporting their efforts to maintain a relationship with families and friends, for example, by finding ways to help with transport, helping them to stay in touch with social and recreational contacts, and helping them to keep links with employment, education, and their local community (National Institute for Health and Care Excellence, 2016).

One such community service is the Individual and Placement Support programme. This has been offered by a range of mental health teams in Britain since 2004 in order to assist mentally ill persons with finding employment (Centre for Mental Health, 2017). The programme is entirely voluntary, in that it is offered only to patients who want to try to find a job. It works by bringing employment specialists – with good contacts with employers – into clinical teams. Together, they provide individualized support for the person and their employer and benefits counselling. While the programme has been implemented somewhat unevenly across the UK, it has proven quite effective in getting participants into jobs (Bond, Drake, and Becker, 2008). Here is how a person suffering from bipolar affective disorder narrates his experience after going through an intensive process with a caseworker helping him to find employment after long spells of unemployment due to his disease:

> Since finding secure employment, I feel like a new person. I hate to sound overconfident or even patronizing to anyone reading this, but I feel like a new man. In ways such as the way I think, act and even the way I carry myself. I can't stress enough how much better I feel having found work. Now I am not shy to talk about my career or even what I do. Whereas before it was very much hiding the fact that I was unemployed, now I look forward to the opportunity to open up about my life. I feel like I walk more confidently and am not shy to speak to strangers, however funny that may seem, I really feel like a happier,

more outward-going positive person. (Miller, Clinton-Davis, and Meegan, 2014, p. 201)

Our point here is not that this personal story is somehow representative of the community services offered to the mentally ill. These services show immense variation in their approach, scope, and efficacy. Our point is rather to illustrate, firstly, that mental health interventions today are not only, or even primarily, about curing disease but about making the mentally ill able to live a more vigorous, happy, and, in this case, more productive life. Secondly, the case illustrates that these interventions do not work through force or coercion but through the freedom of the patient. It is the patient himself who decides to engage in the programme in order to find employment because this will make him happier and able to live a fuller (and wealthier) life.

Not very surprisingly, there are constant concerns over the adequacy of the community services available to the mentally ill. Above all, they are only available to a small proportion of people suffering from enduring mental illness. Moreover, the so-called Out of Area Treatment (OAT), which is primarily placed in independent-sector hospitals, implies that those with the most severe disability are being cared for far away from the community, often at a high cost (Holloway, 2005, p. 1). The inadequacy of existing outpatient services was taken up again in 2012 by the Joint Commissioning Panel for Mental Health (Joint Commissioning Panel for Mental Health, 2012). Based on its analysis of current mental health services, the Commissioning Panel recommended that recovery should be at the centre of all health and social care for people with mental health problems. The services should support users' occupation and work alongside addressing complex medication regimes, physical health, psychological intervention, and everyday living skills (Joint Commissioning Panel for Mental Health, 2012, p. 4). Whether this recommendation has done anything to improve the availability and capacity of community mental health services is unclear. A national survey among NHS employees conducted in 2015 suggests that the number of health staff (nurses) employed in community mental health services has remained constant in the period between 2011 and 2015 (NHS Confederation, Mental Health Network, 2016, p. 8). However, in the same period, the number of nurses was substantially reduced in other psychiatric services, such as hospitals. The same survey found that only 59 per cent of the medical staff working in the mental health services were happy with the standard of service they provided – as compared to a 69 per cent average for all NHS services (NHS Confederation, Mental Health Network, 2016, p. 9). Finally, a recent independent mental health taskforce report, initiated by NHS England, lamented that just half of the Community Mental Health Teams provide a round-the-clock crisis service today (Mental Health Taskforce, 2016, p. 12). The Taskforce urged NHS

England to provide sufficient resources in order to allow the Community Mental Health teams to offer intensive home treatment services around the clock all over England by 2021. These recommendations were apparently accepted by the Secretary of State for Health (Hunt, 2017), and Prime Minister Theresa May announced that public investments in local crisis cafés or havens, which cater to any person suffering from some kind of mental distress, would be doubled (May, 2017).

Conclusion

We have tried to show that recovery has emerged as an increasingly important element in the treatment of mental illness in England since the 1990s. The recovery approach towards mentally ill individuals is found both within and outside the clinical setting. Recovery seems to have gained a foothold within the treatment of mental illness, along with changes in both diagnostic and curative practices. The changing conception of mental illness is perhaps most clearly reflected in the new medical understanding of schizophrenic persons. Both the American and the WHO diagnosis system, DSM and ICD respectively, no longer regard schizophrenia as a wholly chronic disease but now recognize the ability of some patients to recover from the illness.

This changing diagnostic conception is linked to a new approach to cure, by which the aim of becoming completely symptom-free has been replaced by recovery revolving around the ability of the patient to cope with her disease. Accordingly, mental illness is no longer to be cured (only) through the psychiatrist using a curative intervention on the passive object-patient. Rather, recovery seeks to enable the patient to live a fuller and richer life; recovery interventions are clearly linked to interventions and techniques that are believed to nurture the patient's self-steering abilities. Recovery implies that the patient is addressed not only as an expert in his own disease but also as an expert in his own recovery. We thus see an ambiguous relationship between clinical expertise and recovery expertise: the former has paved the way for a clinical argument for recovery and at the same time partially undermined its own expertise in favour of an expertise of experience. In a certain sense, recovery has entailed a democratization of mental health expertise, by which not only the trained psychiatrist but also a wide range of actors, such as psychologists, nurses, social workers, and above all the patient herself, are considered experts.

We have also tried to show that recovery entails the mobilization of social relations and institutions outside the clinical or hospital setting. Thus, under the broad heading of community health services, England has seen the launching of multi-professional teams to assess, plan, and offer effective intervention through individual packages as well as home-based treatment and various outreach activities. Again, this community or psychosocial turn in mental health treatment is linked to the recovery approach because it is part of the same problematization of mental illness. If the problem of the mentally ill is identified as a lack of empowerment, then the cure cannot lie solely within the confines of the clinical or hospital setting but must also include the patient's immediate social environment, such as family relations, friends, the workplace, housing associations, community centres, etc. This entails that it is no longer only the mentally ill person that is the object of biopower, the kind of power seeking to improve the health and vigour of individuals and populations. Biopower has also extended to the patient's surroundings. Thus, in order to be effective, it is necessary to mobilize, structure, and direct the social relations and institutions in which the patient is embedded. The new form of biopower must be extended and multiplied in order to shape the social environment in a way that is conducive to the patient's empowerment and ability to live a fuller life.

Are we then claiming that the emergence of the community approach in the mental health services should be understood as a reflex of the imposition of a more generalized neoliberal discourse? The short answer is no! It may very well be that the community approach to mental health services is in rapport with wider Third Way strategies and the attempts by changing British governments since the 1990s to try to cut public expenditure and delegate responsibility for welfare services to some more or less imaginary communities. However, to reduce the emergence of community psychiatry to some all-pervasive neoliberal ideology misses the point that the emphasis on the role of the extra-clinical setting in treating mental illness hinged on a quite radical shift in the medical conception of mental illness. In other words, the emergence of community psychiatry has its own, distinct genealogy that cannot be reduced to the workings of some master discourse. Yet the point remains that the emergence of this new kind of biopower within mental health seems to have become common sense among health authorities and medical practitioners in the field. Thus, every time this new kind of biopower fails in its own terms either to provide adequate services or to empower patients, the failures are met with calls for the state to invest more to secure the machinations of this power. These persistent calls for more comprehensive and systematic state interventions to mobilize and structure the social relations of the mentally ill also suggest that classical liberal concerns over the dangers of excessive state interventions seem to play a very limited role – if any – in contemporary debates over how best to handle mental illness. In a society (in)famous for its concerns over excessive state interventions, it does seem puzzling that few if any seem to question the moral good of the current doxa: state support and orchestration of community health services is good, more of the same is better.

6

Promoting recovery in Denmark

In 2001, the Danish Prime Minister, Poul Nyrup Rasmussen, gave a speech to the Danish counties at the twenty-fifth anniversary conference celebrating psychiatry's placement within the counties.[1] In the speech, he emphasized the importance of a recovery approach:

> [T]he road to recovery – to recovery from one's illness – is activity and clever conversations. The path away from a deadlock is to have alternatives to the ambivalence, the doubt and the lack of self-esteem. (Statsministeriet, 2001)

The same year, a joint principle programme by both the Ministry of Health and the Ministry of Social Affairs paved the way for recovery to become the official approach in psychiatric treatment. The programme was a central reference when parliament decided in 2001 that recovery should be a core element in treating mentally ill and socially vulnerable individuals (Bertelsen, Harboe, Jeppesen, Jølberg, and Lundum, 2011, p. 10). The programme documentation reads:

> The concept of recovery addresses a systematic attempt to consider the options for a coherent treatment for mentally ill individuals, which also includes the possibility to leave the treatment and social support efforts offered. (Sundhedsministeriet and Socialministeriet, 2001, p. 18)

Hence, in 2001 recovery was explicitly introduced within psychiatric treatment in Denmark (Kromayer, 2003, p. 12), and was to be the guiding principle for treating both the mentally ill as well as socially exposed individuals (Bertelsen et al., 2011).

This chapter examines political rationalities, expertise, and techniques of government involved in the emergence and implementation of recovery in Denmark. As in the previous chapter, we focus on how recovery as a technology of treating mentally ill patients is linked to interventions in their social environment and their everyday lives.

Our overall argument in this chapter is that recovery as a government technology unfolds right between the reciprocally depended practices of what Foucault refers to as government of others and government of the self. Moreover, expertise in recovery is partially held by a health professional whose professionality comes down to being a coach for hopes, dreams, and individual transformation; expertise in recovery is also held by citizens or citizen in constant self-reflection through which their lived life, experiences as a patient, hopes, and dreams are formulated and, concurrently, taken at face value as means for a recovery transformation. It is in the merging of the expertise of individual transformation and the expertise of experience that recovery, both as a means and end, operates as a government technology.

The chapter unfolds in the following way: firstly we single out a few historical events that, in our opinion, show a resemblance to recovery as it is promoted within a Danish setting. Secondly, we offer insight into how recovery has been promoted as an extra-clinical approach to mental illness, followed by an illustration of what may be considered a medico-clinical break with the concept of the chronic psychiatric patient. Accordingly, the chapter provides some examples of recovery efforts launched by the National Board of Health and the Board of Social Affairs at the regional and municipal levels. Finally, the chapter examines how recovery has shaped the relationship between government and self-government, adding further validity to our point, namely to place recovery within a broader analytics of power, as operating through and by virtue of constructive liberalism and vitalism.

Historical antecedents

Recovery's emphasis on the subjective capacities of the patient in her healing process is not an entirely new phenomenon in Danish psychiatric history. In 1930, a debate took place in the weekly medical journal *Ugeskrift for læger* over the term inferiority and the role attributed to the patient's subjective attitudes. Dr Paul Rubow argued that the increase use of 'inferiority' as designating an inner state in the individual, i.e. a feeling of inferiority, was highly problematic (Rubow, 1930, p. 110). Rubow's critique was supported by the medical psychologist Oluf Brüel, who warned against notions such as the 'inferiority complex', denoting a subjective state of mind (Brüel, 1930a). Rubow and Brüel were equally concerned by what they identified as a tendency within medicine to rely on subjective matters, such as an individual's own sense of inadequacy. Medicine, they argued, should instead be based on purely objective judgments, and accordingly, inferiority was to be applied to someone who, in the view of normal members of society, was of lower worth or socially inadequate

(Brüel, 1930b, 1930c, 1930d). Dr Lis Jacobsen supported Brüel and Rubow's point. She blamed psychoanalysis for the inappropriate use of inferiority as an emotional condition (Jacobsen, 1930, p. 1183) and advocated for the term to express a medical diagnosis of the absence of a particular quality (Jacobsen, 1930, p. 1184).

The correspondence summarized above illustrates a crucial question regarding the ends and means of psychiatry: should experts focus on the objective observation of illness from a merely medico-clinical and biological standpoint or are they placed as mediators between objective observations and a patient's subjective attitudes or feelings pertaining to her own illness and health? By ascertaining the difference between defining or objectifying certain individuals as *being* inferior and individuals *feeling* inferior, the debate anticipates the introduction of subjectivity – feelings and self-reflection – as a medical concern. The correspondence in that way illustrates that psychiatry was on the verge of a transformation towards taking into account subjectivity as both a means and end of health; this transformation shows some resemblance to the so-called moral treatment in the nineteenth century.

Inspired by William Tuke and the York Retreat's moral treatment in England, as well as Phillippe Pinel in France (Møllerhøj, 2008, p. 58), moral treatment in Denmark was advocated by Harald Selmer, who was the chief physician at the asylum Jyske Asyl (near Aarhus) during the end of the nineteenth and the beginning of the twentieth century (Møllerhøj, 2008, p. 50), and by Christian Geill, who was the chief physician at the asylum Viborg-anstalten in the same period (Møllerhøj, 2008, p. 51). Selmer found that mentally ill patients ought to be isolated in asylums, far away from the deteriorating influence of the exterior world. According to Selmer, moral treatment was a matter of inciting reflection, discipline, and reason within the patient (Selmer, 1846, pp. 51–52, 56–59). Christian Geill, too, emphasized the necessity of placing the mentally ill patients in secluded asylums, where they would be given the best conditions for recovery (Geill, 1895, pp. 4–5). He regarded moral treatment as a balancing act between freedom and discipline: the restriction of freedom following admission to an asylum ought to be minimized and economized for the purpose of fostering discipline and a work ethic within the patient (Geill, 1895, p. 5). Moreover, the patients ought to be met with compassion as their illness caused them to be unhappy (Geill, 1895, p. 6). Geill supported a so-called *open door system*, by which patients were given a much freedom as possible, while at the same time being disciplined. Unlike medical treatment, Geill argued, freedom and discipline required an individualized approach, by which each patient's characteristics, and the nature of their illness, were accurately determined (Geill, 1895, pp. 42–43).

Moral treatment, as exemplified by the above, was a matter of indirectly influencing the patient towards sanity by addressing both her work ethic (i.e. disciplining her) and her inner compass and sense of responsibility. In this setting we are far away from the self-reflecting techniques at stake in today's recovery approach. Yet we do see that self-steering capacities were regarded as important: the patient is not merely addressed as an insane and doomed individual, out of reach, but is considered a being who can potentially develop into a sane person. As Jette Møllerhøj argues, moral treatment was a kind of psychological swaying, in which the internalization of a disciplining norm was at stake (Møllerhøj, 2008, pp. 58, 60). The term moral here alludes to the soul, the psyche (Møllerhøj, 2008, p. 58). Thus, moral treatment was not to be understood as moralization as such but rather as indirect influence through encouragement and suitable compensations (Kragh, 2008, pp. 102–103). Accordingly, work was considered a central means of cure, in that it could strengthen the patient's self and consciousness (Kragh, 2008, p. 103).

While a sense of the patient's inner reality was merely touched upon in the previous example of moral treatment, in the twentieth century psychology made its claim not only on psychiatry but also on medicine as such. Likewise, the Danish psychiatrist Paul Reiter, in his book on psychotherapeutic techniques, insisted on regarding psychotherapy as a medical treatment of disease through influence on the psyche. Without the help of psychotherapy, Reiter continued, medicine, gynaecology, surgery, and psychiatry would lose their efficacy (Reiter, 1950, p. 10).

Psychological techniques, also referred to as mental hygiene, expanded well beyond the psychiatric practice and clinical setting in Denmark during the mid-twentieth century (T. Hansen, 2008, p. 75). One member of the Association for Mental Hygiene, Ove Lundbye, argued that everywhere where there is contact between human beings, lies a mental hygienic task (Lundbye, 1953, p. 69). In particular the spread of neuroses was considered a central factor in the endorsement of psychological techniques (T. Hansen, 2008, p. 75), which earnestly tapped into ideas of self-reflection and self-steering capacities. As Reiter explains, the cause of suffering is the individual's lack of opportunity to realize himself, his wishes, and his needs (Reiter, 1950, p. 22). Reiter then listed the various elements of psychotherapy: confession, psychotherapeutic interview, instruction, persuasion, awake suggestion, relaxation, psychagogy, autogenetic training, hypnosis, psychoanalysis, narco-synthesis, hypnoanalysis, group therapy, and psycho drama (Reiter, 1950, p. 24). What characterizes most of these techniques is that they address and seek to promote a self-reflective individual, furthering the individual's ability to know herself, understand her psychology, analyse herself, and, accordingly, treat herself. The psychiatrist Thorkil Vangaard explicitly referred to the influence of Freud's psychotherapy within psychiatric treatment. He found it just as scientifically valid as any other psychiatric specialty and referred to the International Psychoanalytical Association as the justification for promoting psychotherapy as a scientific practice (Vangaard, 1955). Other psychiatrists were not so convinced about the merits of psychoanalysis, though they acknowledged its value with regard to the treatment of neuroses (Geert-Jørgensen, 1963, pp. 51–53).

In short, nineteenth-century moral treatment and mid-twentieth-century psychotherapy constitute two quite different approaches to human individuality: while the former seeks to promote self-discipline among the patients treated in the asylums, psychotherapy is a technique centred on self-reflection – within or beyond the confines of psychiatric institutions or clinics. The point is that with the advent of psychotherapy the patient can and should reflect upon herself not only within but also outside the strict psychiatric setting.

An extra-clinical approach

Like England, Denmark has experienced a general move away from a chronicity paradigm, which is first and foremost characterized as a break with the conception of mental illness as a static condition, to a more dynamic and recovery-orientated paradigm. Recovery-orientation is related to a split between a biomedical approach on the one hand and a therapeutic approach on the other, with an emphasis on recovery as a process towards more and more independence and empowerment rather than recovery as actual cure (Topor, 2005, pp. 2–3; Aarhus Kommune, 2007, p. 7; Implement Consulting Group, 2014, p. 21).

A person with a schizophrenic diagnosis epitomizes this break: once considered a sufferer of a serious chronic mental illness, the schizophrenic is now considered amenable to recovery (LAP, 2010, p. 3). Accordingly, recovery may entail being socially recovered: a situation in which the patient has been empowered to handle her symptoms in a way that allows her to lead a more satisfying and productive life. This type of recovery is attained by approximately 35 per cent of those with a schizophrenic diagnosis. Recovery can also be associated with full recovery, that is, living a life without symptoms. This type of recovery, according to the National Board of Social Affairs, is attained by approximately 25 per cent of those with a schizophrenic diagnosis (Socialstyrelsen, 2013, p. 4).

As a fervent advocate of recovery, Swedish psychologist Alain Topor has been a key source of inspiration to the Danish mental health services (Borg, Bengt, and Stenhammer, 2013; Det fælleskommunale sundhedssekretariat, 2014; L. Pedersen and Andreassen, 2015). Topor, too, identifies schizophrenia as the archetypical diagnosis bound to a notion of chronicity and argues for a break with a medico-clinical approach to the disease. This is the case with regard to the disease's duration, course, and organic cause as well as the symptoms, which include an irreversible intellectual and emotional transformation as well as an attack on individual identity (Topor, 2003, pp. 29, 31). The problem with the diagnostic criteria, according to Topor, is the lack of a clear division between organic and psychosocial aspects of the disease, i.e. the aetiology of the diagnosis and the presumably chronic path of the disease (Topor, 2003, p. 33). Moreover, the length of hospitalization has also been considered an indicator of chronicity, and patients with schizophrenia are often committed to hospital for long periods (Topor, 2003, p. 36). Topor argues that instead of looking for schizophrenia's roots in individual characteristics, be they biological or psychological, we should pay attention to the patient's social life, including damage through institutionalization and stigmatization. Topor argues that research shows that patients, after being discharged from hospital, in many cases did not display clinical symptoms but nevertheless had difficulties adapting to society and their local community. Hence, a social criterion is called for, according to Topor (Topor, 2003, pp. 37–38), by which increased quality of life has taken over the notion of cure (Topor, 2003, p. 29). Chronicity is strongly associated with diagnosis, but the notion of recovery is a move away from the strict emphasis on diagnoses (Topor, 2003, p. 30). Topor refers to the concept of nursing, i.e. developing a set of positive values: cure, remission, adaption, improvement, and recovery. Topor's argument illustrates how the promotion of recovery entails a break with a medico-clinical focus on illness and cure, and, instead emphasizes a psychosocial focus on quality of life and recovery. It also illustrates how the patient is freed from a strict categorization along the lines of a diagnosis to be placed within a somewhat blurry category *between* illness and cure, *between* impairment and quality of life: the patient might be schizophrenic, but she is nevertheless freed from the negatively loaded association following the diagnosis. Moreover, she might be negatively affected by her illness and yet be able to overcome the heavy burden of disease through her hopes and dreams and thereby increase her quality of life.

Today, mental recovery efforts in Denmark are no longer restricted to schizophrenic patients but are used with people with almost all psychiatric diagnoses. In Psychiatric Services for the Capital Region, for instance, recovery is the explicit aim and means for all psychiatric patients under treatment, whether inpatients or outpatients:

> The visions for future psychiatry take into consideration that the patient is at the centre of attention, and this is why the recovery idea is essential. We use methods and means which supports the recovery process of each individual. The message 'you can recover' is the essence of recovery, and therefore we are focusing on hope, possibilities and empowerment. (Region Hovedstadens Psykiatri, 2016)

Accordingly, today's mental health services propose more or less the same set of therapeutic strategies and techniques in the pursuit of recovery regardless of the diagnosis. Uffe Ladefoged, a social psychiatry manager in Northern Jutland, lists a number of elements that are all related to a recovery approach: explicit personal goals in the treatment of psychiatric patients, patient participation for inpatients, a planned release from hospital, recovery mentors, so-called Shared Decision Making, open dialogue, and a strategy for user participation (Ladefoged, 2014). In addition, the National Board of Social Affairs lists the following stimulating measures for recovery to take place: a feeling of belongingness to a community, hope and optimism, creating a positive identity, meaning, and empowerment (Socialstyrelsen, 2013, p. 10).

Recovery may emphasize a process of increasing the individual's independence from psychiatric treatment and social efforts. However, it may also entail an expansion of the relatively narrow medico-clinical gaze on the psychiatric patient to include a wide range of psychological, economic, and social aspects of her life. The former resembles individual recovery, which was promoted by Bennet and Lieberman in the US in the 1960s and which asserts that an individual with a decreased psychic functioning level can increase his mental abilities. The latter approach, on the other hand, is in alignment with Anthony's idea that an individual with decreased psychic functioning can learn to work and achieve a successful life with as little intervention as possible (see Wilken and den Holländer, 2008, pp. 25–26, 108; Eplov, Korsbek, Petersen, and Olander, 2010, pp. 25–26). The first understanding is concerned with developing individual coping skills; the second is inspired by self-help trends in the 1970s (Wilken and den Holländer, 2008, p. 41) and with developing support systems in the community (Eplov et al., 2010, pp. 25–26). This division reflects recovery's intimate relationship with rehabilitation: while recovery primarily concerns means towards recovery from mental illness, rehabilitation primarily deals with the activation of social efforts – i.e. a supportive social environment to enable the individual's recovery process. It also illustrates that mental recovery approaches may be aligned both with laissez-faire or limited state intervention, the central aim being government through self-government and with an extensive state intervention in order to create a more or less dense institutional and social network that may assist the recovery of the individual patient.

Recovery and rehabilitation found a new, and to some extent more challenging, relationship with the structural reform of the Danish public sector, implemented in 2007. The reform divided psychiatric efforts into treatment, on the one hand, and preventive health, social support, and health promotion, on the other. The former is mainly a regional task, whereas prevention and promotion are municipal tasks. Hence, the five regions are in charge of the treatment of those individuals whose mental suffering is considered serious enough to be enrolled in the mental health system. The 98 municipalities offer social support, housing, and the like for patients who have finished treatment but are still considered in need of public support.

On the face of it, it may seem as though the structural reform has impaired the wider spread of a recovery approach by its separation of clinical mental health from social psychiatry and the social aspects of mental health services. However, this administrative gap between the mental health services and the social services has been bridged, at least partially, in the sense that the mental health services have adopted a recovery approach, in which primarily recovery techniques aimed at individual patients are used. The municipalities – being in charge of social support for the mentally ill – have adopted a recovery approach more in line with rehabilitation, in which the activation of the social environment is at the forefront of their services. Finally, efforts have been made to support a strong collaboration between the two sectors. Shared Care, for instance, was launched as a collaborative project between Psychiatric Services for the Capital Region and seven municipalities in the western part of Copenhagen (Rådgivende Sociologer, 2014).

In summary, in line with developments in England, recovery in Denmark breaks with the notion of certain psychiatric illnesses as a chronic state. Schizophrenia reflects this change of perception, changing its status from being incurable to being either partly or wholly curable. At the same time, the schizophrenic patient is often cited by health authorities as an example of how to approach recovery, namely less as a question of removing all symptoms and more as a process towards more and more independence and empowerment. Moreover, recovery in Denmark has expanded to all areas of psychiatry, including regional psychiatric treatment and municipal social-psychiatric support. In fact, the introduction of the structural reform in 2007, despite the clear distinction between treatment and social support, seems to have paved the way for kind of recovery that is intimately linked to rehabilitation.

Recovery projects

Danish recovery efforts are fully integrated into both regional and municipal mental health services. Promoting recovery as an explicit goal and means that most psychiatric efforts imply more or less directly a recovery approach. Initiatives by the National Board of Health and the Ministry of Health have published a number of documents in which recovery is promoted. Additionally, a number of semi-autonomous associations, such as the Danish Association for Psychosocial Rehabilitation (Dansk Selskab for psykosocial rehabilitering) and Knowledge Centre for Social

Psychiatry (Videnscenter for Socialpsykiatri) – which are partially funded by the state – have not only placed recovery on the mental health agenda but also established a direct link between recovery efforts and psychosocial efforts targeting mentally ill individuals.

Many of the projects within the Danish mental health system do not have an explicit recovery approach but nevertheless incorporate a general mix of psychosocial methods within the framework of recovery. The techniques used are varied and to some extent even contradictory. Still, they are related through joint means and end: self-reflection and empowerment.

A research consultant at Psychiatric Services for the Capital Region, Lene Eplov, argued that psychotherapeutic methods in general can be seen as associated with recovery, including cognitive therapy, psychodynamic therapy, psychoeducation, and family interventions (Eplov et al., 2010, pp. 61–62, 71–72). Also, the Shared Care approach is a framework for doing recovery (Wilken and den Hollænder, 2008, p. 108). Shared Care is a model for collaboration between regions and municipalities as well as private actors, with the purpose of increasing the wellbeing of psychiatric patients. The model has been implemented in a number of regions (Rådgivende Sociologer, 2014).

Moreover, the National Board of Health's so-called *satspulje* from 2014 to 2017 aimed at promoting outpatient crisis teams for psychiatric patients in the regional psychiatry service (Sundhedsstyrelsen, 2014a). The Psychiatric Frederiksberg Centre, which is part of the Psychiatric Services for the Capital Region, has also promoted crisis teams doing outpatient treatment in the patient's home or immediate environment as an alternative to inpatient treatment (Region Hovedstadens Psykiatri, 2015a) Both projects are inspired by Crisis Assessment and Treatment Teams (CAT-teams), which have been promoted in Melbourne, Australia since the 1990s (Johnson, 2013) and later in England (National Audit Office, 2014).

Likewise, the Centre Region (Region Midt) in Jutland has promoted a number of initiatives that can be more or less directly related to recovery. In 2008, the Psychiatry House was opened in Silkeborg, offering urgent treatment 24/7 as well as training in social skills. The opening of the house was linked to a collaborative project with eight municipalities in the Centre Region aimed at investigating to what extent social skill training in groups can enhance the recovery process. The project has been evaluated and the conclusion was clear: those participating in social skills training became better at participating in social settings and were better at taking care of themselves, increasing the expectations of what can be changed (Ankersen et al., 2014).

SIND, equivalent to the British MIND, opened an activity centre in which patients work towards increasing their potential through art and creativity, a process referred to as creative recovery (Nielsen, 2006b). In Aarhus municipality, recovery orientation has been emphasized as part of social psychiatry (Aarhus Kommune, 2007), incorporating therapeutic techniques that are person-centred and empowerment-orientated (Aarhus Kommune, 2007, p. 13). The latter is associated with developing self-confidence, overcoming feelings of powerlessness and gaining opportunities for change and control of the future (Aarhus Kommune, 2007, p. 15). A key notion in this regard is to find meaning and develop coping strategies (Aarhus Kommune, 2007, pp. 14–15).

OPUS is a multidisciplinary outreach treatment team within Psychiatric Services for the Capital Region directed at young patients with emerging psychosis or an illness within the schizophrenia spectrum (Nordentoft and Iversen, 2010, p. 132). OPUS started as an independent research project in 1998, and today it covers 13 teams in total (Nordentoft and Iversen, 2010, p. 132). The treatment lasts two years, and OPUS consists of a team of psychiatrists, nurses, social counsellors, occupational therapists, and psychologists (Nordentoft and Iversen, 2010, p. 132). The focus is on regaining or increasing the patient's functional level as well as providing focused occupational projects (Nordentoft and Iversen, 2010, pp. 134–136).

To promote recovery in Psychiatric Services for the Capital Region, the Competence Centre for Rehabilitation and Recovery was formed, which, among other initiatives, launched a School for Recovery. The 2016 programme states that the courses are developed in collaboration between former or current psychiatry service users and professionals; each workshop provides both a teacher with user background and a professional as well as a user relative representative (Region Hovedstadens Psykiatri, 2016, p. 5). For patients, the courses offer help in discovering their personal journey towards recovery as an individual transformation process, by gaining insight into their physical and psychological wellbeing; by identifying goals, ambitions and dreams; by being in the company of other course members; and, finally, by experiencing a supportive and learning environment. For relatives, the courses provide an insight into how to help themselves and how to support others in their recovery process. The courses provide an opportunity for professionals to gain more knowledge about recovery, to gain experience of being schooled together with patients and relatives, and to share and learn from others (Region Hovedstadens Psykiatri, 2016, p. 6). The courses include 'five ways to a good life' (Region Hovedstadens Psykiatri, 2016, p. 8), a theme concerning how to live with bipolar affective disorder; how to live with psychosis and schizophrenia (Region Hovedstadens Psykiatri, 2016, p. 9); how to find a community and move on (Region Hovedstadens Psykiatri, 2016, p. 10), with titles such as 'Common decisions – because the patient too is an expert', 'Guide to a good everyday life' (Region Hovedstadens Psykiatri, 2016, p. 11), 'Introduction to mindfulness', 'Personal dreams and goals' (Region Hovedstadens Psykiatri, 2016, p. 12); and 'Recovery – a life in change' (Region Hovedstadens Psykiatri, 2016, p. 13).

Alongside regional recovery projects, various municipalities have adopted a recovery approach within their social-psychiatric offers. Among Copenhagen's municipal social services is the social-psychiatric residence centre Lindegården, which supports citizens who suffer from a psychiatric illness and are considered unable to fully take care of themselves. Lindegården's recovery approach centres on residents' rights, respect, care, and collaboration (Center Lindegården, 2017). Although residents at the centre are considered unable to take care of themselves, a primary aim at the residential centre is to strengthen their abilities to do so (Center Lindegården, 2017, 2011, p. 7). Related to this aim is Lindegården's focus on making residents more active. Residents will be helped to seek regular jobs locally or within Copenhagen municipality and, concurrently, work at Lindegården. The work offered to the residents ranges from growing vegetables (Center Lindegården, 2017, p. 8), cooking together with the employees (Center Lindegården, 2017, p. 7), cleaning, caretaking (Center Lindegården, 2017, p. 16), working in the café (Center Lindegården, 2017, p. 13) to working at the commercial department. The work here includes packaging, mounting, labelling, and sorting, and the residents are given a salary (Center Lindegården, 2017, p. 12). It is stressed that all activities are to be aligned with the way the residents wish to live their lives, their hopes, and their dreams (Center Lindegården, 2017, p. 18).

In brief, the public mental health system in Denmark has developed a number of interventions and projects informed by the recovery approach. Some projects draw on the recovery approach, such as the OPUS team for young people with emerging psychosis. Other projects engage in collaborative strategies, adopting integrated solutions that involve regions, municipalities, and private initiatives and that seek to improve the psychosocial wellbeing of psychiatric patients. Some projects also include psychotherapeutic methods that cannot be directly linked to a recovery approach per se, such as initiatives to increase the self-engagement of psychiatric patients as well as initiatives for outpatient treatment. Yet even these initiatives, which typically take place within the home of the patient, seek to engage relatives and the community in the therapeutic process. The establishment of peer support in most parts of the counties' psychiatric wards, and the relatively high influence of the user associations SIND and LAP, as well as citizens' direct engagement in the implementation of treatment, also reflect that recovery has gained a footing within current mental health treatment.

The self-steering individual

In the following section, we first account for how the patient or user organizations for mentally ill persons, LAP and SIND, have been integrated into the mental health services with a view towards offering treatment along the lines of user orientation. Secondly, we elaborate on the user orientation approach by taking our point of departure from arguments presented by various experts in the treatment of mentally ill individuals. Finally, we look into particular strategies presented by the National Board of Health and the Ministry of Health, which stress user orientation as a central means for recovery. Our point is to draw attention to how user orientation nurtures and gives credence to what may be termed the expertise of experience and thereby paves the way for the patient to embody her mental illness and her recovery at the same time.

The National Association of Present and Former Psychiatry Users (Landsforeningen Af nuværende og tidligere Psykiatribrugere), LAP, has managed to gain strong influence within regional psychiatric services. LAP has particularly advocated for psychiatric patients' rights to take part in decision-making concerning psychiatric treatment. The organization has members connected to the regions' psychiatric services, and they are present when decision-making takes place, participate in conferences, and the like. As argued in one of LAP's articles: the user's will and interests should as far as possible set the point of departure for the efforts provided. If illness, medication, addiction, or other factors hinder this, LAP suggests that a 'life testament' should be considered, in which the user – when in a better state – can formulate his own wishes (E. Olsen, 2016). LAP advocates for psychiatric patients to join the workforce (LAP, 2010). Some articles, as in the case of the work done by Topor for LAP, explicitly argue for a recovery approach, underscoring user inclusion and empowerment as central aspects of recovery: 'Hope gives birth to a will to change things' (Topor, 2005, p. 8). This argument is based on the assumption that even the most severely afflicted patient has relatively benign periods. The rationale of recovery, Topor asserts, is to enable people with a mental illness to develop their own method, follow their own path, and form their own understanding of how to cope with their disease (Topor, 2005, p. 19).

Like LAP, the national user and relatives' association SIND (equivalent to the British MIND) has for a number of years promoted the idea that mentally ill patients should have more influence on their own treatment. More recently, SIND's 2015 plan of action placed recovery as one of its five key points (SIND, 2015). SIND is represented on the government's Psychiatry Committee and has a number of SIND ambassadors working to promote its cause, among them former Prime Minister Poul Nyrup

Rasmussen and Crown Princess Mary, who is SIND's official sponsor (SIND, 2016).

A number of psychiatric units in the Capital Region systematically integrate user accounts and patient experiences into treatment as an active resource for recovery. The patient is seen as holding unique knowledge about her own experiences and life situation and is used as a role model and living proof of the possibility of recovery (Region Hovedstadens Psykiatri, 2014, pp. 3, 17). These so-called 'recovery mentors' (Region Hovedstadens Psykiatri, 2014, 2015b, 2015c), also referred to as 'peer supporters' or 'peer workers' (Olesen, 2015, p. 21), typically work part-time within the mental health services (Region Hovedstadens Psykiatri, 2014, p. 15; Tønder, 2014). Those psychiatric organizations that directly include peer support are more likely to achieve recovery among users (Kromayer, 2003, p. 14). In this way, the professional worker is acknowledging the user's life world and experiences as a central means for recovery (Wilken and den Holländer, 2008, p. 29).

Among other initiatives, the Competence Centre for Rehabilitation and Recovery has developed a recovery mentor service. The service is offered to patients on selected wards, giving them the opportunity to talk to a person who has a mental illness and has been admitted to a psychiatric ward. The mentor, who is hired by Psychiatric Services for the Capital Region, provides hope and general knowledge about recovery, drawing explicitly from his own experience (Kompetencecenter for Rehabilitering og Recovery, 2016). Moreover, the Centre has promoted a number of activities with a view toward enhancing the patient's expertise of experience. As stated in an article by the Centre: 'It is a new way of thinking ...: Can personal experiences become equalized with scientific knowledge?' (*Tidsskriftet Outsideren*, 2016). The Competence Centre takes the promotion of the expertise of experience to its full potential. Those working at the Centre are both employees and individuals suffering from a mental illness, and the courses are equally for professionals and patients, all asked to open up and step out of their usual roles (Kompetencecenter for Rehabilitering og Recovery, 2016).

Psychiatric Services for the Capital Region has outlined five elements for recovery to take place: belongingness, hope, identity, meaningfulness, and empowerment (Region Hovedstadens Psykiatri, 2015d). The idea is for the patient to become in tune with the treatment she receives by actively writing down what she hopes to gain after the treatment (Region Hovedstadens Psykiatri, 2015e). Moreover, recovery is about creating a new self-image (Region Hovedstadens Psykiatri, 2014, p. 2). A central focus is on user-orientated treatment, emphasizing the patient's achievement of a meaningful life (Dall, 2013, p. 23). Likewise, the National Board of Health has actively promoted peer support. In 2014, the Board created a pool for financing peer support within municipalities, regions, and user organizations (Sundhedsstyrelsen, 2014b). Hence, patient participation in treatment and the creation of personal goals by and with the patient are central means of recovery (Region Hovedstadens Psykiatri, 2015c).

The recovery approach is person-centred (Slade, 2013, p. 4), emphasizing the need to be on an individual journey (LAP, 2005, p. 19; Slade, 2013, p. 5) through which the person defines her own recovery (Socialstyrelsen, 2013, p. 4; Region Hovedstadens Psykiatri, 2015d), and thereby increases her self-esteem and possibility of becoming empowered (Socialstyrelsen, 2013, p. 10). An empowering setting is promoted both via individual empowerment and motivation (Slade, 2013, pp. 25, 26, 27) and by nurturing a space for active citizenship (Socialstyrelsen, 2013, p. 12). The empowering setting may include particular social efforts – i.e. rehabilitation – which support recovery, such as providing courses aimed at integrating the patient into the workforce, courses in social skills, psycho-education and mindfulness (Socialstyrelsen, 2013, pp. 13, 14). The promotion of an empowering setting entails a number of elements, which are usually provided to the patients by asking them to relate to the following: their dreams, their goals, and the difference between the two (Region Hovedstadens Psykiatri, 2015f); the articulation of short-term and long-term goals; considering how to move on in life; and reflecting on which path is the proper one to follow (Region Hovedstadens Psykiatri, 2015f). The promotion of an empowering setting is further underlined by inviting patients to actively relate to the role of the environment, including family relations (Region Hovedstadens Psykiatri, 2015g). The idea is to develop and validate personal meaning (Slade, 2013, p. 18) and to foster personal responsibility and self-management skills (Slade, 2013, p. 25; Region Hovedstadens Psykiatri, 2015g).

Closely related to the focus on recovery as an individual process is the notion of recovery as in fact an existential process of becoming closer to one's core being, which includes the user's 'whole life' (Dall, 2013, p. 7). Rather than being a search for truth, it is a question of looking for meaning (LAP, 2005, p. 1; Topor, 2005, p. 18). The idea is to avoid placing too much emphasis on the patient's diagnosis but instead to take into account the patient as an individual (Kromayer, 2003, p. 12), and thereby allow her to reclaim her self-esteem (Kromayer, 2003, p. 13). Rather than a static condition, recovery is seen as a process towards regaining more self-functioning and becoming part of society (Wilken and den Holländer, 2008, p. 26). In general, the promotion of recovery includes the (re-)establishment of a positive identity (Socialstyrelsen, 2013, p. 10) and socializing efforts to reinforce the feeling of belonging (Socialstyrelsen, 2013, p. 10).

So, what does developing one's own method imply for therapeutic interventions? Topor argues that self-reflection methods within psychiatric treatment often have a tendency to become integrated within the patient, instead of her finding her own methods. This, for example, is the case with psychodynamic therapeutic treatment, where installing insights within the patient in terms of her psychic condition, at the same time, according to Topor, incorporates the psychiatric system's norms within the patient (Topor, 2003, p. 48). An alternative version is one where the patient reconquers her claim to independence without being prone to normalization (Topor, 2003, p. 53). This individual journey is seen as a process towards improvement. The first step is to overcome rigidity, or in other words to acknowledge and accept the mental illness and find hope and motivation to change the condition. The intermediate step is discovering and developing self-empowerment by reclaiming one's self. Finally, the last step concerns improving one's quality of life by striving towards increasing wellbeing and a higher level of functioning (Topor, 2003, p. 125). Referring to Goffmann, Topor asserts that the chronically ill individual has taken over the psychiatrist's definition of herself (Topor, 2003, pp. 40–41). The emphasis here is placed on the necessity of viewing recovery as a path, which the person herself feels is right for her (Torpor, 2005, p. 6). While the notion of cure is strictly connected to symptoms and the removal of symptoms, rehabilitation focuses on individual functioning and development. In both cases, professionals are key actors. Recovery, on the other hand, places the individual within a broader life perspective, where an individual's own efforts and network efforts are included (Topor, 2003, p. 41).

Conclusion

This chapter has demonstrated how recovery is promoted in Denmark as a means for empowerment through and by virtue of the patient, her whole life, her feelings, and her opinions. The empowerment aspect of recovery is linked to the critique of former, presumably medico-clinical, approaches towards mentally ill patients, primarily schizophrenic patients, which considered such patients to be incurable. We have also tried to show that recovery taps into a liberal norm of self-government, nurtured both through techniques of self-realization and by activating a social support system. The former is reflected in the clinical, psychological, and social efforts aimed at the patient's hopes and dreams of the future with a view toward installing hope for recovery, and the social support system is reflected in the wide range of extra-clinical setting, such as the family, social relations, the local community and the workplace. The separation of social services from treatment services, which followed from the 2007 structural reform, has challenged the implementation of recovery strategies and programmes as they hinge on a close link between these two spheres. Yet we also saw the launch of a wide range of collaborative projects, such as Shared Care, which seek to integrate a social aspect in the treatment of patients and thereby tie a strong knot between recovery and rehabilitation.

We examined some of the recovery projects to show how recovery is put into practice both by regions and municipalities. We found that, although the National Board of Health has not launched any recovery strategies since the beginning of the millennium, recovery has indeed found footing within the Danish mental health services, which stress extra-clinical factors, downplay clinical factors, and thereby question, if not undermine, the formerly strict division between the patient and the professional. As an effect of recovery's promotion of empowerment techniques, the patient is credited with an expertise in experience that is valued higher than traditional medico-clinical expertise. In this new expertise of experience, social and psychological expertise are mutually at work, nurturing the patient's hopes and dreams to come to the fore and be articulated. However, the patient's expertise can only be activated as long as she actively takes part in the process.

In the case of England, we have shown how some private organizations, such as the Royal College of Psychiatrists, manage to distinguish their work from the work of the mental health services in general. Moreover, they have managed to place recovery and rehabilitation on the agenda long before it was adopted by the NHS as an official strategy. In Denmark user organizations like LAP and SIND have managed to make their cause known to the broad public, and their agenda correlates more or less perfectly with the agenda set by the National Board of Health. This is especially clear with regard to both parties' emphasis on the use of peers in mental health treatment. Recovery has been adopted within all areas of mental health services and is practised both at the regional and the municipal level. The question remains whether this somewhat frictionless relationship between private associations and the mental health services, in the sense that recovery has been fully adopted on both stands, comes at a price; in other words, whether it has compromised the progressive potential of recovery.

While the use of recovery in England and Denmark differs in several respects, we also find a number of similarities when gauged through the conceptual framework of governmentality and biopower. Firstly, in both countries, recovery is promoted as an appreciative expertise within a facilitating environment aimed at nurturing positive change with regard to the mentally ill person. It seems as though transformation towards recovery can only occur in a positive and all-embracing manner. What characterizes this appreciative and positive attitude? By nurturing the individual's hopes and dreams, professionals draw attention to a potential future that might occur through a constant transformation. Transformation is key here. In contrast, stagnation is not an option of any kind. More generally, problematizations of the blessings of the ever-changing ethos of self-government are seen as a liability to appreciation and thereby positive transformation. On this score, recovery empowers the patient along the lines of raising her awareness of her *potential* being, *possible* future, and *imaginable* life. We have characterized this attitude as optimistic vitalism, as it promotes life and living in a positive and appreciative way.

That said, the promotion of vitalism in this setting is contradictory. The individual – i.e. the patient – is addressed as someone who can either stagnate into her illness or transform towards recovery by strengthening her self-reflective and self-steering capacities. Passivity thus has to be overcome through an active choice towards recovery. However, the kind of vitalism that recovery seeks to activate is not that of the living body, but rather the self-reflecting mind. If ever the mentally ill patient was considered a lewd and sexually uncontrollable being, whose bodily activities were regarded as too vital, acting out her rampant vitality uncontrollably, this is no longer the case. The patient of today's recovery is urged to engage in a constant act of self-reflection and transformation, setting her mind towards the *possibility* of living more fully, dreaming of and hoping for something else, as long as it is different from today. Vitalism then is promoted in relation to transformation per se, i.e. transformation is for the better – not as the promotion of life and living as such.

Secondly, this self-reflective and self-steering individual, who is addressed through recovery, is an ethical being at its fullest, as she is engaged in a constant self-subjectifying act. Accordingly, the health professionals and social workers are facilitators of recovery, fostering a positive environment, which enables a transformation to take place along the lines of the individual's ethical workings upon herself. We identify this kind of amelioration of an ethical being as constructive neoliberalism, as it essentially relies on the self-steering capacities of the individual. The extra-clinical setting promoted along with recovery is first and foremost a setting that psychologically and socially supports the individual's ability to govern herself. Bearing in mind Foucault's identification of the relationship between the government of others and the government of oneself, we may even go as far as to argue that government of others relies solely on the government of oneself. Put differently, it is as if government along the lines of recovery justifies itself only in so far as it is linked to self-government. And this seems to be the core of a constructive neoliberalism: if neoliberalism has puzzled over the question of how to govern without cohesion, the answer for constructive neoliberalism is to govern only through self-government.

Note

1 After the structural reform of 2007 counties no longer exist and regions have taken over responsibility for mental health services.

Conclusion

In the preceding chapters, we have tried to show that contemporary health politics in England and Denmark has undergone a substantial mutation since the 1980s. Based on our analysis of obesity control and mental recovery, we found that health promotion strategies and interventions have supplemented and partially recast earlier curative and preventive approaches in both England and Denmark. On the one hand, it is clear that curative approaches, which focus on the identification, treatment, and elimination of clinically specified illness, and physical prevention, which focuses on the provision of clean water, the management of sewage and waste, and food safety regulations, both continue to play a fundamental role in public health politics. On the other hand, it seems clear, at least in the areas of obesity control and mental recovery, that health promotion strategies seeking to augment the productivity and vigour of individuals and the population through a wide range of institutional, psychological, and socializing interventions have grown substantially since the 1980s.

Obesity control

The emergence of obesity as an object of health promotion in England and Denmark displays a number of similarities. In both countries, political concerns over body weight emerged during the early twentieth century in tandem with eugenic discourses about the quality of the population or stock. While the main concern was with underweight individuals and inadequate nutrition among the poor classes, being overweight also gained increasing attention. In England, obesity was mainly taken as a sign of the degeneration of the British race precipitated by the growth of an urban middle class taking up sedentary occupations (office work). This concern informed the formation of the body culture movement in the 1930s. While obesity received rather modest attention in Denmark at that time, the weakening of physical stamina and ensuing moral decay was the object of intense debate, which informed the rise of a highly popular and well-organized gymnastics movement. In both England and Denmark, the body culture and gymnastics movements respectively were mainly driven and orchestrated by private individuals and organizations, with the state's role mainly limited to providing a certain level of financial support for these activities.

With the decline of eugenics – both in its negative and its positive versions – obesity would not receive much attention for the next half-century. But when obesity came back on to the political agenda, it did so with a remarkable force in both England and Denmark. During the 1980s, obesity was rearticulated as a political problem when medical knowledge pointed to the relationship between obesity and diabetes, cardiovascular diseases, and various forms of cancer. While a preventive and integrated approach inspired by the WHO's Health for All strategy was suggested, very little concerted action was actually taken until the late 1990s. The main intervention took the form of improved information (product labelling and information campaigns) in order to appeal to the rational and responsible liberal subject.

From the late 1990s, two general strategies were employed in both countries in the attempt to control obesity: individualizing and environmental. The individualizing interventions worked to single out those deemed at risk. In principle, all citizens are at risk; however, in practice, people with a high BMI and children of parents with a high BMI were targets of the most intense attention for a variety of medical, pedagogic, and psychological interventions. One of the most spectacular examples of individualizing interventions are the so-called fat camps where obese children and – in increasingly more cases – adults are trained in the art of governing themselves in a healthy manner. Here the focus is not only on dieting and physical exercise but also on social activities in order to develop the self-esteem of the obese. While there was much talk during the early 2010s on the potential of nudging techniques particularly in England, this has so far played a relatively limited role, mostly due to the practical problems of adopting viable solutions.

The second strategy implied a wide set of interventions targeting the social environment of essentially all citizens – in England mainly referred to as 'community', in Denmark mainly referred to as 'society'. It was imagined that community empowerment – in various forms – would strengthen the opportunity for citizens to choose a healthy lifestyle. This entailed the development of a quite comprehensive apparatus of central and local authorities teaming up with a wide range of voluntary organizations and to some extent also for-profit organizations in order to create an institutional environment encouraging more people to adopt a healthier lifestyle. In

England, such programmes have involved local government, community centres, schools, workplaces, and various companies under the heading of joined-up government (Blair) or Big Society (Cameron). In Denmark, the structural reform of 2007 implied that municipalities stepped up their interventions and systematically started to link up with families, schools, workplaces, gymnastics and sports clubs to create an institutional web that strongly urges obese persons to reconsider and change their lifestyle. This relatively clear centralization of the orchestration of obesity control interventions in Denmark (with the municipalities) seems to constitute an important difference from England. Here the NHS and to some extent the Local Government Association may have acted as the hub of such programmes. However, most strategies have delegated responsibilities to other local authorities and to private actors. Another difference has to do with the relatively popular and highly organized Danish gymnastics and sports movement, which decided shortly before the structural reform in 2007 to work closely with municipalities in the area of health promotion, including obesity control. This seems to have created a more densely institutionalized web of obesity control programmes and services than the one found in England.

Obesity control via these two health promotion strategies has not been very successful when judged by its own terms. In both England and Denmark, the prevalence of overweight and obese people kept increasing between the 1980s and around 2010, when the growth rate was reduced in England (Public Health England, 2016) and halted in Denmark (Sundhedsstyrelsen, 2014c). Thus, on the face of it, the Danish obesity control apparatus seems to have been slightly more effective than the British one, perhaps because of the more fully institutionalized web described above. At any rate, the limited effectiveness of obesity control interventions in both England and Denmark has not led to any political calls for the abandonment of this approach. In fact, the quest for empowering communities and their citizens has only increased. Thus, changing English and Danish governments since the late 1990s have relied not only on appealing to the rational citizen by way of product labelling and information campaigns but also on direct interventions targeting communities and individual obese persons. The contemporary obesity apparatus is expanding in a seemingly limitless fashion not only because it identifies and targets 'patients before their time' (B. Evans and Colls, 2011) but also because its failure is taken as an argument for the need for further development and expansion. The homology with Foucault's analysis of the (failing) disciplinary and rehabilitating strategy informing prison reforms in the early nineteenth century seems rather obvious (Foucault, 1977a).

We think that our analysis of obesity control proves two common understandings of contemporary (neoliberal) health policies wrong or, at the very least, problematic. On the one hand, the argument that the new preventive health policies evolving around the notion of risk tend to individualize and privatize the responsibility for poor health or for the risk of poor health (for an overview, Rockhill, 2001) is a gross exaggeration, at least in the case of obesity control. We have shown that state and local authorities in both England and Denmark have intervened extensively in the area of obesity since the late 1990s. Yes, medical experts and many left-wing politicians would like more interventions and bemoan the budget cuts in this area during the 2010s in England. But that is not to say that public health interventions in this area have become less ambitious or withdrawn. Also, one of, it not the most, important strategies pursued since the 1990s targets not individuals but the community. The invention of the community as a sphere of moral rectitude and a site of intervention has proved crucial to obesity control.

On the other hand, we also disagree with those who argue that obesity control is above all an objectifying and repressive apparatus (Gard and Wright, 2005; B. Evans and Colls, 2009). It may very well be that the label of obesity may in some cases be stigmatizing. Yet our analysis suggests that the kind of medical power pursued in contemporary obesity policies works not so much through objectification and repression but above all through voluntary self-subjectification. True, the medical discourses around obesity objectify the obese. Also, the kind of self-subjectification endorsed by the many interventions is a highly structured and relatively narrow one. The obese and the non-obese alike are constantly reminded that they should reflect on their choice of diet, their everyday physical conduct, their social relations, and thus their self-esteem. Yet the point is exactly that the interventions are not trying to impose a disciplinary scheme on a passive target group. Rather they entail a form of power that works by structuring the institutionalized space of self-government. People must actively govern themselves according to the regulatory ideals of optimistic vitalism if they are going to avoid obesity and lead a productive and vigorous life.

Mental recovery

Mental recovery with its emphasis on the subjectivity of the patient only emerged in its current form at the end of the twentieth century, though certain elements of this approach are already found in the treatment of mentally ill people both in England and Denmark in the nineteenth century. In the early nineteenth century, so-called moral treatment was introduced in England and in Denmark. What characterized moral treatment in both cases was the idea of addressing the patient as potentially curable – and thereby also capable of making morally correct choices. This early treatment worked by instilling in the patient a sense of responsibility while at the same time disciplining her. Moral treatment thus contains the early seeds of self-steering techniques as a therapeutic means towards sanity. From the early twentieth century we find a similar emphasis on the self-steering capacities of the individual patient through psychoanalytic treatment where the patient is encouraged to actively take part in her own cure. Although psychoanalysis had only a limited influence on the treatment of mentally ill patients, its techniques of self-reflection and active participation gained footing in patient treatment both inside and outside the mental institutions.

Recovery in England and Denmark has developed differently, though we also find similar themes and techniques. In both countries, recovery found a voice as part of an anti-psychiatric, or more precisely an anti-clinical critique of the treatment of mentally ill patients, which first and foremost manifested itself in a change of attitude towards schizophrenic patients, who for the most part had been considered incurable by definition. Recovery offers a move away from the chronicity paradigm and an emphasis on empowering the patient by addressing her self-steering capacities, while at the same time activating a social support system outside of the institution, in the community and the family. In England, private associations have paved the way for a recovery approach, which was further supported by the development of systematized clinical guidelines. In England, one of the strongest advocates for recovery has operated outside the public health system but nevertheless supported by it. The Royal College of Psychiatrists in London has been active in promoting social psychiatry and emphasizes rehabilitation as being intimately linked to recovery. Although the Royal College of Psychiatrists is an independent private organization, whose purpose is to set a standard and to promote high-quality mental health services, it has largely managed to place recovery on the agenda and has strongly influenced the recovery promoted by the Department of Health. Another important private actor is the National Collaborating Centre for Mental Health. This organization has been commissioned by the NHS and NICE to develop and secure evidence-based treatment. These factors all tap into a community-based focus vis-à-vis the recovery approach, i.e. rehabilitation. The Royal College of Psychiatrists, for instance, initiated a number of rehabilitation services that were supported by the NHS. While the NHS has not developed a national strategy for rehabilitation, it has supported the development of services offered by local government and communities.

In Denmark, on the other hand, recovery has been an explicit aim and goal of the Ministry of Health and the mental health services offered by the counties (now regions). A central inspiration has been the Swede Alain Topor, and his emphasis on empowerment has influenced the official policies. Although health policies and social policies are divided into a regional and a municipal task respectively, recovery techniques have managed to gain footing in both areas. Outpatient treatment, collaborative strategies for the integration of regional, municipal and private initiatives, and the establishment of peer support within psychiatric wards as well as the integration of user associations in the decision-making process of treatment, all give credence to a recovery approach.

In short, the promotion of recovery first and foremost operates in an extra-clinical setting by which the local community and the family are activated as a social support system. At the same time, recovery places attention on the individual patient and though empowerment and therapeutic techniques offers her a positive attitude towards her illness, allowing the illness to become an instigator for a positive transformation towards recovery.

The specificity of health promotion

We should be wary of exaggerating the novelty of health promotion in the same way that we should not fall prey to the cynical and facile claim that nothing has really changed in the governing of public health. Obviously, political concerns over body weight and mental health have a longstanding history in the West. We have also indicated that both phenomena have been the object of systematic state interventions at least since the beginning of the twentieth century in both England and Denmark. The biopolitical concern with body weight and mental health has not only been addressed through curative approaches but also through a number of preventive approaches, which culminated with the eugenics movement in the first half of the twentieth century. Thus, preventive interventions directly intervening in the lives of individuals in the name of the population's productivity and vigour are clearly not new. Viewed at this fairly abstract level, health promotion seems to amount to little more than a tiny permutation of the kind of biopower emerging in most Western European states' around the beginning of the nineteenth century.

Yet we find that health promotion does constitute a significant novelty. While we think that health promotion is a form of biopower in the sense of state-initiated and -financed interventions seeking to ensure the population's health and vigour, it implies several novelties with substantial political implications for those subjected to it. The novelty of health promotion rests not so much with its attention to prevention but with its way of governing through the freedom of individuals, communities, and other parts of civil society. True, health promotion certainly contains a strong element of prevention. Yet the policies, programmes, and techniques employed under the heading of health promotion work above all through the subjectivity of the governed groups, not through coercion, as was the case with negative eugenics. Also, the preventive strategies to boost hygiene by modifying the physical environment adopted in England and Denmark from around the end of the nineteenth century rarely if ever entailed any form of coercion, like contemporary health promotion. Yet again, voluntarism and freedom of choice is not the same as governing through freedom and the subjectivity of the target group. The health reformers of the late nineteenth and early twentieth century may have been concerned with the physical quality and mental ability of citizens, but the reforms they proposed never required that these citizens reflect and act upon themselves in order to choose a healthier mode of conduct or, as it came to be called, lifestyle. Nor did it occur to them that the surroundings in which citizens lived could matter in other terms beyond the purely physical and biomedical. It is only with health promotion that the environment or the community takes on an institutional and normative importance for guiding the citizen's choice of lifestyle.

More precisely, the current quest for health promotion can be specified according to the techniques of power that it employs, the types of knowledge that enable it, and the political rationalities that inform it. Health promotion hinges on *techniques of power* that seek to empower and mobilize the resources of the people that it targets. The power techniques of health promotion may be divided into two broad groups, namely individualizing and socializing techniques. The *individualizing techniques* seek to single out and promote the health of the ill person, the person at risk of becoming ill, or, more broadly, the person at risk of becoming less vigorous. In the area of obesity control, we have seen the proliferation of tailored fitness programmes for the obese, boot camps, dietary courses teaching nutrition knowledge and cookery skills, and psychological counselling seeking to boost the self-esteem of the obese. In the area of mental recovery, the individualizing techniques seek to install within the individual self-awareness and empowerment, along the lines of hopes, dreams, and positive expectations for the future. Yet the hopes and dreams primarily allude to the quest for living a normal life and having a job. These individualizing interventions have received much academic and some political attention and have often been criticized by left-wingers for delegating the responsibility of poor health to the individual and for justifying budget cuts in public health services. While this may have been the case, particularly during the recent British Coalition government led by David Cameron, this should not make us overlook the fact that public health authorities and services in both countries have invested substantial resources in programmes that seek to enable people to assume a higher degree of responsibility for, or, more precisely, to be better able to govern, their own health. Moreover, the individualizing responsibility critique tends to overlook the other group of power techniques at play, namely socializing techniques.

Both in the area of obesity control and mental recovery, health promotion interventions have systematically tried to invoke and mobilize the *institutional environment* of the obese and the mentally ill in order to enhance their capacities to better take care of themselves. These interventions seek to create a dense network between families, friends, peers, schools, workplaces, companies, sports clubs, and community centres in ways that will help the obese adopt a healthier lifestyle and enable the mentally ill person to better cope with his clinical symptoms and live a fuller life. This governmentalization of communities or, more broadly, civil society in order to promote the health of the population has for some reason received rather scant attention from critical scholars. We find this neglect curious. In contrast to individualizing interventions, in which people can always decline to participate in a given programme, it is much more difficult to say no to living in an environment thoroughly institutionalized by networks and norms of the correct lifestyle, be that in terms of your body weight or your mental health.

Health promotion is also characteristic and partially novel in terms of the *bodies of expert knowledge* that inform it. Unlike curative approaches, which rely almost exclusively on biomedical knowledge, and physical preventive interventions, which rely on hygiene and epidemiological knowledge, health promotion relies on a wide mix of expert knowledges: biomedical, hygienic, epidemiological, psychological, pedagogical, social work, sociological, and public administration. Firstly, the bodies of knowledge enabling curative and physical prevention interventions work primarily through objectification. They seek to define, diagnose, circumscribe, classify, and quantify the object of illness and the spread of disease with a view towards curing or even preventing it from arising. These forms of knowledge are essentially unable to work through the subjectivity or the freedom of people. While health promotion interventions certainly also rely on the objectifying capacities of biomedicine, hygiene, and epidemiological knowledge, they differ from earlier, public health approaches by interventions working through the subjectivity of people. It is above all pedagogy and psychology that help problematize the obese and the mentally ill in terms of a lack of capacity or power to govern themselves in a way that would allow them to live a more vigorous life, and it is these two bodies of knowledge that provide the various approaches, procedures, methods, and techniques for encouraging the individual to conduct himself differently. And it is above all social work, sociology, and public administration expertise that point to the detrimental effects of weak social ties with family and peers, lack of social capital, inadequate coordination, and insufficient collaboration between public organizations. And it is these three bodies of knowledge that more or less directly inform the many interventions seeking to solidify social ties with family and peers, rebuild community bonds, develop effective, joined-up government, and nurture networks between frontline health services and the various private groups and citizens. These forms of knowledge target not the subjectivity of the individual but the empowering and self-governing capacities of the institutional environments that will support the obese in choosing a healthier lifestyle and will assist the mentally ill individual in his recovery activities.

Finally, health promotion is characterized by its specific *political rationalities*. While it remains part of a biopolitical enterprise that started around two centuries ago in most Western European states, including England and Denmark, the political rationality of health promotion is characterized by a particular form of *optimistic vitalism* or optimizing vitalism. This vitalism rests on the dictum that everyone should live a life that is as vigorous and productive as possible: citizens should govern themselves accordingly, and public authorities should stimulate this particular exercise of freedom. It is this vitalism that is expressed in the WHO's Health for All strategy from the mid-1980s and in more or less articulate forms in the concrete interventions targeting the obese and the mentally ill in England and Denmark since around 1990. One characteristic of this form of vitalism is that it applies to each and every member of the population, as argued above. Moreover, this vitalism does not hinge on normalization. The rationale of obesity control is not to normalize individuals according to some statistically calculated normal person, for no other reason than fat is the new normal. Instead the aspiration is to make citizens adopt a lifestyle, a way of conducting themselves, in which they reflect on their diet and physical activity in their everyday life in ways that will enhance their productivity and vitality. Rather than normalization, health promotion works by structuring a particular field of ethics, a space within which the citizen is expected to reflect more or less constantly upon their own health and wellbeing.

Apart from believing that every citizen always can and should try to improve the productivity and vigour of his life, optimistic vitalism also regards the state as responsible for securing the conditions allowing and stimulating citizens' attempts to engage in actions enhancing their vigour. This dimension is correlated with a particular form of neoliberalism that may be labelled constructivist neoliberalism (Triantafillou, 2017). In contrast to the kind of (critical) neoliberalism that takes the market as its benchmark for designing, assessing, and criticizing government interventions, constructivist neoliberalism takes the self-governing capacities of individuals, groups, communities, and networks as its object. Whereas critical neoliberalism is fundamentally sceptical of interventions launched by public authorities, as they always run the risk of ignoring the preferences of individuals and thwart the exchange of information about such preferences through the market, constructivist neoliberalism is concerned with how the state may construct markets, communities, public service delivery, and citizens in ways that enhance their self-governing capacities. Even if it agrees with its critical sibling that the state should be very careful of intervening directly into the lives of citizens, communities, and markets, it does not rest on the axiom that markets and other social phenomena are given and that they will always function better if the state keeps away. Rather, it asks: to what extent does this citizen, community, market, public service delivery, or company govern itself in a socially desirable way? And how can the state create and improve the conditions that will make these actors exercise their freedom in a way that it is even closer to socially desirable norms. In the case of health promotion, these norms are propagating the constant attention to and improvement of the productivity and vigour of the life of individuals and state populations.

The analytical value of the notions of biopower and governmentality

Foucault's concepts of biopower and governmentality are both relevant to understanding contemporary health promotion interventions in liberal democracies. The term biopower is useful in grasping the way in which health promotion innovates but ultimately retains the state's concern with the biological quality of the population inhabiting its territory. While the exercise of biopower in both England and Denmark has undergone substantial changes since its emergence in the nineteenth century, we find that the term biopower is still useful in creating a space for critically analysing the ways in which state power in liberal democracies is concerned, perhaps more than ever, with the vigour of populations. The constant political debates and ensuing interventions sparked by the comparative epidemiological surveys of longevity, illness rates, and obesity rates testify to the persistent concern of states with the vigour of the populations inhabiting their territory. Today, these surveys do not only feed into assessments of the relative vigour of populations inhabiting state territories vis-à-vis other states (Frandsen and Triantafillou, 2011). They also inform debates about the relative efficacy of public health interventions. It is these epidemiological surveys, combined with health expenditure accounts, that make countries like the US and Britain seem highly ineffective in their ways of ensuring longevity and controlling obesity. In turn, these surveys and accounts are used to substantiate claims for making the state intervene more effectively in the lives of its citizens.

To understand why biopower does not revert to more direct forms of interventions targeting individual behaviour, the notion of governmentality is useful. As we suggested above, health promotion seems to be informed by constructivist neoliberalism. This is a liberal governmentality in that it more or less systematically assumes the existence of and works through the freedom of citizens and civil society (N. Rose, 1999). It is this liberal concern with the freedom of individuals, communities, and private organizations that problematizes paternalist schemes like nudging and rejects updated versions of eugenics regulating the procreation of the population by way of new genetic mapping technologies. By the same token, constructivist neoliberalism is not just some updated version of social welfarism through which illness is addressed in terms of adequate collective insurance systems and the availability of medical services. According to social welfarism, the kind of governmentality informing a wide range of social welfare reforms all over the Western world from the late nineteenth century to around the 1970s, the problem of poor health is above all one of lacking economic income and having inadequate physical amenities and environments. Accordingly, the solution is to provide better access to health services through collective insurance and intervene through urban planning, housing regulations, and other infrastructure to create a healthy environment for all social groups. None of these interventions requires or seeks to invoke the freedom or the self-steering capacities of citizens. Finally, if constructivist neoliberalism is concerned with the freedom of those over or through whom power is exercised, we should note that it differs importantly from other forms of liberalism.

The term governmentality is particularly useful in order to clear a space for analysing the often multiple and contradictory rationalities at stake in contemporary attempts to govern the health and vigour of individuals and populations. Many of the disputes around health promotions have to do with the different rationalities of government at play in the politics of health. For many politicians and academics of some kind of leftist orientation, health promotion is a problematic endeavour to the extent that it may be used to justify the withdrawal of the responsibility of the state to provide adequate health services and ensure proper housing and working conditions. Drawing more or less directly on social welfarist rationalities, this critique does not believe that the problem lies with inadequate self-esteem, weak social ties, or inactive communities but with constant budget cuts in the public health sector, insufficient funding for affordable and sanitary housing, and the haphazard implementation and enforcement of workplace regulations jeopardizing health. Conversely, classical liberal rationalities have been invoked to problematize contemporary proposals for prohibiting smoking, strictly regulating alcohol consumption, and forcing obese parents to change their diet under the threat of removing their children. As indicated by our studies, these other political rationalities seem to be less influential than constructivist neoliberalism, but they are clearly part of the contemporary debates on how best to control obesity and handle mental illness.

The problematic character of health promotion and optimistic vitalism

We have tried to address the optimistic vitalism underpinning contemporary health promotion not as a theory, an ethos, or a *pathos* to be either lamented or celebrated but as an empirical phenomenon to be critically analysed. As we argued in the Introduction, we find several debates about the utility and validity of vitalism as a theoretical framework for understanding life or as an ethos for the conduct of life, but very few that have examined vitalism as a contemporary element of biopower. This may be because health promotion really has nothing to do with vitalism. However, we think that vitalism, in the sense of aspirations for increasing the productivity and vigour of individuals and even populations, is key to contemporary health promotion. The lack of research into this area is particularly disconcerting because health promotion proposes a form of vitalism, an optimistic or optimizing vitalism, that has no immanent political limitations.

From the point of view of wanting to maximize freedom and allow for the widest possible reversibility of existing power relations, health promotion (and the vitalism it implies) is deeply problematic because of its grand and seemingly unlimited ambitions of promoting the health of all by way of governing and mobilizing society at large. Of course, we should be careful not to exaggerate the influence of health promotion vis-à-vis other health strategies. And we should be particularly careful not to overlook the fact that health promotion does allow and even stimulate new forms of freedom whereby patients, citizens, communities, and other subjects can govern their health in novel ways that they find desirable. Yet health promotion is not only generating new forms of freedom; it is also actively discouraging other forms. It discourages any form of conduct that is regarded as risky or unhealthy. In the area of obesity control, people with a high BMI and who are therefore, objectively speaking, overweight or obese are seen as people unable to govern themselves adequately and in need of intervention – whether they like it or not. In fact, people who are most resistant to receiving help are seen as those with the toughest problem, because they obviously do not recognize that they have a problem. Thus, the key indicator for legitimizing health promotion interventions is not body weight but the person's attitude and thus his subjectivity. It is true that not all contemporary health promotion techniques work through subjectivity involving personal self-reflection. Above all, the technique of nudging promises to provide weight reduction by various non-conscious nudges, but the bulk of medical and social expertise still relies on the assumption that lasting weight loss can only be generated by inducing a mental change in the obese person, i.e. the ways in which he conceives of himself, his body, and his self-esteem, and the ways in which he interacts with family, friends, colleagues, etc. In brief, the obese person should only change not his behaviour but his subjectivity. It is simply not acceptable to engage in forms of freedom that do not include the constant reflection on eating habits, physical exercise and routines, and rapport with other people affecting your self-esteem.

In the area of mental recovery, the patient who merely accepts his mental illness, and the disabilities following the illness, would be considered passive and so obstructing his own potential to change for the better. To put it differently, the freedom to stay fixed and inflexible in terms of one's illness is not an option. Even on its own terms, health promotion is questionable, as it tends to focus rather narrowly on charging individuals and communities with the responsibility for changing lifestyles. In the case of obesity, numerous studies have documented the statistical correlation between excessive weight and low levels of education and income. Yet contemporary health promotion does not imply any attempt to increase educational attainment or equalize economic incomes. What is particularly disconcerting is that public authorities, medical experts, and various empowerment engineers have so few qualms about intervening so extensively and quite directly into the lives of citizens and their surroundings. While classical liberalism's focus on the space of privacy was loaded with all kind of governmental ambitions, such as securing an order based on property rights and law-abiding citizens, at least it entailed a certain moderation of state interventions in people's lives. This inhibition seems be increasingly undermined in the name of public health promotion.

Bibliography

Aarhus Kommune. (2007). *Styrket Recovery-orientering i den psykosociale rehabilitering*. Aarhus: Socialforvaltningen, Århus Kommune.

Ackerknecht, E. (1968). *A Short History of Medicine*. Baltimore, MD: Johns Hopkins University Press.

Ahlstrand, L., and Pihl, N. (2010). Sundheds- social- og handlingspolitik. In L. Eplov, L. K. Falgaard, L. Petersen, and M. Olander (eds), *Psykiatrisk og psykosocial rehabilitering – en recoveryorienteret tilgang*. Copenhagen: Munkgaard Danmark, pp. 179–191.

Ankersen, P. V., Dürr, D. W., Møller, T. D., Madsen S. M., and Væggemose, U. (2014). *Døgndækkende psykiatrisk hjemmebehandling – et alternativ til akut indlæggelse?* Viborg: Folkesundhed og Kvalitetsudvikling, Region Midtjylland.

Anthony, W. A. (1993). Recovery from mental illness: the guiding vision of the mental health service system in the 1990s. *Psychosocial Rehabilitation Journal*, 16(4): 11–23.

Anthony, W. A. (2004). The recovery effect. *Psychiatric Rehabilitation Journal*, 27(4): 303–304.

Anthony, W. A., and Farkas, M. (1982). A client outcome planning model for assessing psychiatric rehabilitation interventions. *Schizophrenia Bulletin*, 8(1): 13–38.

Antonovsky, A. (1996). The salutogenic model as a theory to guide health promotion. *Health Promotion International*, 11(1): 11–18.

Appleby, L. (2007). *Mental Health Ten Years On: Progress on Mental Health Reform*. London: Department of Health.

Armstrong, D. (2002). *A New History of Identity: A Sociology of Medical Knowledge*. Basingstoke: Palgrave Macmillan.

Ayo, N. (2012). Understanding health promotion in a neoliberal climate and the making of health conscious citizens. *Critical Public Health*, 22(1): 99–105.

Baggott, R. (2011). *Public Health. Policy and Politics*. 2nd edn. Basingstoke: Palgrave Macmillan.

Baggott, R. (2013). *Partnerships for Public Health and Well-Being: Policy and Practice*. Basingstoke: Palgrave Macmillan.

Bambra, C., Fox, D., and Scott-Samuel, A. (2005). Towards a politics of health. *Health Promotion International*, 20(2): 187–193.

Barber, M. E. (2012). Recovery as the new medical model of psychiatry. *Psychiatric Services*, 63(3): 277–279.
BBC News. (2007). Obesity 'as bad as climate risk'. news.bbc.co.uk/2/hi/health/7043639.stm.
Beattie, A. (1991). Knowledge and control in health promotion. In J. Gabe, M. Calnan, and M. Bury (eds), *The Sociology of the Health Service*. London: Routledge.
Beck, U., and Beck-Gernsheim, E. (2002). *Individualization*. London: Sage.
Behavioural Insights Team. (2013). *Applying Behavioural Insights to Organ Donation*. London: Cabinet Office Behavioural Insights Team. www.behaviouralinsights.co.uk/trial-results/applying-.
Behavioural Insights Team. (2016). Health. www.behaviouralinsights.co.uk/category/health/.
Bender, E. (2012). People in recovery are key part of psychiatry dept. staff. *Psychiatric News*, 47(9): 14–15.
Bercovitz, K. L. (1998). Canada's Active Living policy: a critical analysis. *Health Promotion International*, 13(4): 319–328.
Bergson, H. (1911). *Creative Evolution*. New York: Henry Holt and Co.
Bertelsen, P., Harboe, L., Jeppesen, P. P., Jølberg, R., and Lundum F. (2011). Social og personlig recovery. *Psykolog Nyt*, 16: 10–13.
Blank, R. H., and Burau, V. (2014). *Comparative Health Policy*. 4th edn. Basingstoke: Palgrave Macmillan.
Bond, G., Drake, R., and Becker, D. (2008). An update on randomised controlled trials of evidence-based supported employment. *Psychiatric Rehabilitation Journal*, 31(4): 280–290.
Bonde, H. (1991). *Mandighed og sport*. Odense: Odense Universitetsforlag.
Borg, M., Bengt, K., and Stenhammer, A. (2013). *Recoveryorienterede praksisser. En systematisk videnssamling*. Report no. 4/3013. Copenhagen: Dansk Selskab for Psykosocial Rehabilitering.
Braidotti, R. (2002). *Metamorphoses: Towards a Materialist Theory of Becoming*. Cambridge: Polity Press.
Braveman, P., Egerter, S., and Williams, D. R. (2011). The social determinants of health: coming of age. *Annual Review of Public Health*, 32(1): 381–398. doi.org/10.1146/annurev-publhealth-031210–101218.
Brend, W. (1917). *Health and the State*. London: Constable and Co.
Breton, E., and de Leeuw, E. (2011). Theories of the policy process in health promotion research: a review. *Health Promotion International*, 26(1): 82–90.
British Nutrition Foundation. (2012). Behaviour change and obesity. www.nutrition.org.uk/healthyliving/behaviour/behaviourchange.html.
British Psychoanalytic Council. (2017). British Psychoanalytic Council: about us. www.bpc.org.uk/about-us (accessed 14 March 2017).
Brown, B. J., and Baker, S. (2012). *Responsible Citizens: Individuals, Health and Policy under Neoliberalism*. London: Anthem Press.
Brown, P. (2016). Bariatric surgery rarely performed in Britain. Better access could cut long-term burden on patients. *Medpage Today*. www.medpagetoday.com/endocrinology/obesity/57856.
Brownson, R. C., Baker, E. A., Leet, T. L., Gillespie, K. N., and True, W. R. (2011). *Evidence-Based Public Health*. Oxford: Oxford University Press.

Brüel, O. (1930a). Mindreværdighed. Correspondence. *Ugeskrift for læger*, 45(6 November): 1055.
Brüel, O. (1930b). Mindreværdighed. Correspondence. *Ugeskrift for læger*, 49(6 December): 1165.
Brüel, O. (1930c). Mindreværdighed: En sproglig-terminologisk bemærkning. Correspondence. *Ugeskrift for læger*, 42(16 October): 996.
Brüel, O. (1930d). Socialinsufficiens – socialinsufficient. Correspondence. *Ugeskrift for læger*, 46(13 November): 1075.
Bryant, T. (2002). Role of knowledge in public health and health promotion policy change. *Health Promotion International*, 17(1): 89–98.
Bunton, R., Nettleton, S., and Burrows, R. (1995). *The Sociology of Health Promotion: Critical Analyses of Consumption, Lifestyle and Risk*. London: Routledge.
Butland, B., Jebb, S., Kopelman, P., McPherson, K., Thomas, S., Mardell, J., and Parry, V. (2007). *Foresight. Tackling Obesities: Future Choices – Project Report*. London: Department of Innovation, Universities and Skills. www.gov.uk/government/uploads/system/uploads/attachment_data/file/287937/07–1184x-tackling-obesities-future-choices-report.pdf.
Cabinet Office. (2011). *Behavioural Insights Team. Annual Update 2010–11*. London: Cabinet Office. www.cabinetoffice.gov.uk/sites/default/files/resources/Behaviour-Change-Insight-Team-Annual-Update_acc.pdf.
Cain, R. (2013). 'This growing genetic disaster': obesogenic mothers, the obesity 'epidemic' and the persistence of eugenics. *Studies in the Maternal*, 5(2): 1–24.
Campos, P. (2004). *The Obesity Myth: Why America's Obsession with Weight is Hazardous to Your Health*. New York: Gotham.
Canguilhem, G. (1991). *The Normal and the Pathological*. New York: Zone Books.
Canguilhem, G. (1994). *A Vital Rationalist*. New York: Zone Books.
Castel, R., Castel, F., and Lovell, A. (1982). *The Psychiatric Society*. New York: Columbia University Press.
Center Lindegården. (2011). Velkommen til Center Lindegården. Information til nye beboere og deres pårørende. http://docplayer.dk/1515477-Velkommen-til-center-lindegaarden.html (accessed 1 February 2018).
Center Lindegården. (2017). Velkommen: Velkommen til Center Lindegården – et socialpsykiatrisk bocenter. https://centerlindegaarden.kk.dk/ (accessed 1 February 2018).
Chiu, L. F. (2003). *Application and Management of the Community Health Educator Model. A Handbook for Practitioners*. Leeds: Nuffield Institute for Health.
Christiansen, N. S., Holmberg, T., Hærvig, K. K., Christensen, A. L., and Rod, M. H. (2015). *Kortlægning: Kommunernes arbejde med implementering af Sundhedsstyrelsens forebyggelsespakker 2015. Udvikling i arbejdet fra 2013–2015*. Copenhagen: Center for Interventionsforskning, Statens Institut for Folkesundhed, Syddansk Universitet.
Christiansen, N. S., Pedersen, C. H., Holt, D. H., Holmberg, T., Christensen, A. I., and Rod, M. H. (2014). *Kortlægning. Kommunernes arbejde med implementering af Sundhedsstyrelsens forebyggelsespakker. Midtvejsrapport*. Copenhagen: Center for Interventionsforskning, Statens Institut for Folkesundhed, Syddansk Universitet.

Christiansen, P. M., and Nørgaard, A. S. (2002). *Faste forhold – flygtige forbindelser. Stat og interesseorganisationer i Danmark i det 20. århundrede.* Aarhus: Aarhus Universitetsforlag.

Clarke, A. E., Shim, J. K., Mamo, L., Fosket, J. R., and Fishman, J. R. (2003). Biomedicalization: technological transformations of health, illness, and U.S. biomedicine. *American Sociological Review*, 68: 161–194.

Coffey, J., Budgeon, S., and Cahill, H. (eds) (2016). *Learning Bodies: The Body in Youth and Childhood Studies.* Singapore: Springer.

Conrad, P. (2007). *The Medicalization of Society.* Baltimore, MD: Johns Hopkins University Press.

Corbett, S., and Walker, A. (2012). The Big Society: back to the future. *Political Quarterly*, 83(3): 487–493.

Corbin, A. (1986). *The Foul and the Fragrant: Odour and the French Social Imagination.* Cambridge, MA: Harvard University Press.

Craig, T. (2006). What is psychiatric rehabilitation? In G. Roberts, S. Davenport, F. Holloway, and T. Tattan (eds), *Enabling Recovery: The Principles and Practice of Rehabilitation Psychiatry.* Trowbridge: Cromwell Press, pp. 3–18.

Crawshaw, P. (2012). Governing at a distance: social marketing and the (bio) politics of responsibility. *Social Science and Medicine*, 75: 200–207.

Dall, T. (2013). På vej mod en rehabiliterende beskæftigelsesindsats. Om rehabilitering og tværprofessionelt arbejde i de nye reformer på beskæftigelsesområdet. *Uden for nummer. Tidsskrift i forskning og praksis i socialt arbejde*, 26: 4–13.

Danske Gymnastik- og Idrætsforeninger. (2005). *Strategisk samarbejde sikrer idrættens sundhedsprojekter. Nyheder og udspil.* 8 March. www.dgi.dk/arkiv/2005/03/08/strategisk-samarbejde-sikrer-idraettens-sundhedsprojekter.

Danske Gymnastik- og Idrætsforeninger. (2011). *DGI Strategi 2015.* http://e-pages.dk/dgi/547/.

Danske Gymnastik- og Idrætsforeninger. (2013). *DGIs vedtægter af 9. November 2013.* www.dgi.dk/om/fakta/baggrund/vedtaegter.

Danske Gymnastik- og Idrætsforeninger. (2016a). *DGI Sundhedsidræt.* www.dgi.dk/sundhedsidraet/baggrund-for-projektet/.

Danske Gymnastik- og Idrætsforeninger. (2016b). *DGI Certificering: Bliv DGI Børnehave and Vuggestue.* www.dgi.dk/om/samarbejd-med-dgi/kommunesamarbejde/certificering/dgi-vuggestue-boernehave.

Danske Gymnastik- og Idrætsforeninger. (2016c). *DGI Certificering: Bliv DGI Profilskole.* www.dgi.dk/om/samarbejd-med-dgi/kommunesamarbejde/certificering/dgi-profilskole.

Danske Gymnastik- og Idrætsforeninger. (2016d). *Samarbejde i lokalsamfund giver ny motivation.* www.dgi.dk/foreningsledelse/goer-din-forening-bedre/samarbejde-i-lokalsamfund.

Dansk Institut for Klinisk Epidemiologi. (1989). *Udviklingen i sundhedstilstanden i 80erne.* Copenhagen: DIKE.

Dansk Institut for Klinisk Epidemiologi. (1993). *Middellevetid og dødelighed. En analyze af dødeligheden i Danmark og nogle europæiske lande, 1950–1990.* Copenhagen: Middellevetidsudvalget.

Dansk Institut for Klinisk Epidemiologi. (1998). *Sund By Netværket. Baggrund, tilblivelse, udvikling og aktiviteter 1988–97.* Copenhagen: DIKE.

Davies, E., Gardner, E., and White, C. E. S. (2015). Childhood obesity. Fit for the future. *Journal of Family Health*, 25(4): 39–42.

Dean, M. (1991). *The Constitution of Poverty: Toward a Genealogy of Liberal Governance*. London: Routledge.

Dean, M. (1994). *Critical and Effective Histories: Foucault's Methods and Historical Sociology*. London: Routledge.

Dean, M. (1995). Governing the unemployed self in an active society. *Economy and Society*, 24(4): 559–583.

Dean, M. (1999). *Governmentality: Power and Rule in Modern Society*. London: Sage.

Deleuze, G. (1988). *Bergsonism*. New York: Zone Books.

Den Korte Avis. (2014). Sådan holdes børns vægt nede med simple midler: Holbæk-læger vækker international opsigt. http://denkorteavis.dk/2014/enkle-regler-hjaelper-born-med-at-holde-vaegttabet/?print.

Dennis, R. (2015). Beyond policy analysis: the raw politics behind opposition to healthy public policy. *Health Promotion International*, 30(2): 380–396.

Department of Health. (1998). *The Health of the Nation – A Policy Assessed*. London: The Stationery Office.

Department of Health. (1999). *A National Service Framework for Mental Health. Modern Standards and Service Models*. London: Department of Health.

Department of Health. (2000). *The Expert Patient. A New Approach to Chronic Disease Management in the 21st Century*. London: Department of Health.

Department of Health. (2001). *The Journey to Recovery – The Government's Vision for Mental Health Care*. London: Department of Health.

Department of Health. (2003). *Annual Report of the Chief Medical Officer 2002: Health Check on the State of the Public Health*. London: Department of Health. www.dh.gov.uk/en/Publicationsandstatistics/Publications/AnnualReports/DH_4006432.

Department of Health. (2004). *Choosing Health: Making Healthier Choices Easier*. London: Department of Health.

Department of Health. (2008). *Healthy Weight, Healthy Lives: A Cross-Government Strategy for England*. London: HMSO.

Department of Health. (2010). *Healthy Lives, Healthy People: Our Strategy for Public Health in England*. London: The Stationery Office.

Department of Health. (2011). *Healthy Lives, Healthy People: A Call to Action on Obesity in England*. London: Department of Health.

Department of Health. (2015a). *Policy Paper. 2010 to 2015 Government Policy: Obesity and Healthy Eating*. London: Department of Health. www.gov.uk/government/publications/2010-to-2015-government-policyobesity-and-healthy-eating/2010-to-2015-government-policy-obesity-and-healthy-eating.

Department of Health. (2015b). *Living Well for Longer: One Year On*. London: Public Health Policy and Strategy Unit, Department of Health.

Department of Health and Social Security. (1977). *Prevention and Health*. London: HMSO.

Dikötter, F. (1998). Race culture: recent perspectives on the history of eugenics. *American Historical Review*, 103(2): 467–478.

Doyal, L., and Pennell, I. (1979). *The Political Economy of Health*. London: Pluto Press.

Drake, R. E., and Whitley, R. (2014). Recovery and severe mental illness: description and analysis. *Canadian Journal of Psychiatry*, 59(5): 236–242.
Dreyfus, H. L., and Rabinow, P. (1982). *Michel Foucault: Beyond Structuralism and Hermeneutics*. London: Harvester Press.
Durkheim, E. (1968). *Suicide: A Study in Sociology*. London: Routledge and Kegan Paul.
Egedal Kommune. (2015). *Holbæk-modellen. Behandling af overvægtige børn og unge*. www.egedalkommune.dk/media/1674164/holb_k-modellen.pdf.
Eggar, G., and Swinburn, B. (2002). Preventative strategies against weight gain and obesity. *Obesity Reviews*, 3: 289–301.
Eplov, L. F., Korsbek, L., Petersen, L., and Olander, M. (2010). *Psykiatrisk og psykosocial rehabilitering – en recoveryorienteret tilgang*. Copenhagen: Munkgaard Danmark.
Ettrup, C., and Olsen, O. (2014). J. P. Müller. In *Dansk Biografisk Leksikon*. Copenhagen: Gyldendal. http://denstoredanske.dk/index.php?sideId=294524.
Evans, B. (2010). Anticipating fatness: childhood, affect and the pre-emptive 'war on obesity'. *Transactions of the Institute of British Geographers*, 35(1): 21–38.
Evans, B., and Colls, R. (2009). Measuring fatness, governing bodies: the spatialities of the body mass index (BMI) in anti-obesity politics. *Antipode*, 41(5): 1051–1083.
Evans, B., and Colls, R. (2011). Doing more good than harm? The absent presence of children's bodies in (anti-) obesity policy. In E. Rich, L. F. Monaghan, and L. Aphramor (eds), *Debating Obesity. Critical Perspectives*. Basingstoke: Palgrave Macmillan, pp. 115–138.
Evans, M. (2014). Mum with NHS gastric band now demands 'fat camp' funding for her 17-stone daughter. *Express*, 28 July.
Faaborg-Midtfyn Kommune. (2013). *Implementering af 3–4-års besøg i Den Kommunale Sundhedstjeneste i Faaborg-Midtfyn Kommune*. Ringe: Faaborg-Midtfyn Kommune.
Det fælleskommunale sundhedssekretariat. (2014). *Kommunernes fælles rolle – udviklingen af det nære sundhedsvæsen på psykiatriområdet. Fælles rammer og målsætninger for kommunerne i hovedstadsregionen*, 24 March. Copenhagen: Det fælleskommunale sundhedssekretariat.
Farrant, W. (1991). Addressing the contradictions: health promotion and community health action in the United Kingdom. *International Journal of Health Services*, 21(3): 423–439.
Fein, O. (1995). The influence of social class on health status: American and British research on health inequalities. *Journal of Internal Medicine*, 10: 577–586.
FitFarms. (2016). About FitFarms. www.fitfarms.co.uk/index.php (accessed 10 January 2017).
Flegal, K. M., Kit, B. K., Orpana, H., and Graubard, B. I. (2013). Association of all-cause mortality with overweight and obesity using standard body mass index categories: a systematic review and meta-analysis. *JAMA*, 309(1): 71–82.
Fleming, P. (2007). Workplaces as settings for public health development. In A. Scriven and S. Garman (eds), *Public Health: Social Context and Action*. London: Open University Press, pp. 166–179.
Fokus-Nyt. (2003). *Kommunestrukturen i et historisk lys*, no. 24, December. Denmark: Fokus.

Foo, L. L., Vijaya, K., Sloan, R. A., and Ling, A. (2013). Obesity prevention and management: Singapore's experience. *Obesity Reviews*, 14(Suppl. 2): 106–113.

Forebyggelseskommissionen. (2009). *Vi kan leve længere og sundere. Forebyggelseskommissionens anbefalinger til en styrket forebyggende indsats.* Copenhagen: Forebyggelseskommissionen.

Forordning om koppevaccination 1810. (2016). Retrieved from *Danmarkshistorien.dk*. Aarhus: Aarhus Universitet, Institut for Kultur og Samfund. http://danmarkshistorien.dk/leksikon-og-kilder/vis/materiale/forordning-om-koppevaccination-1810/.

Foucault, M. (1967). *Madness and Civilization*. London: Routledge.

Foucault, M. (1973). *The Birth of the Clinic*. New York: Vintage Books.

Foucault, M. (1974). *The Archaeology of Knowledge*. London: Tavistock Publications.

Foucault, M. (1977a). *Discipline and Punish: The Birth of the Prison*. London: Penguin Books.

Foucault, M. (1977b). Nietzsche, genealogy, history. In D. F. Bouchard (ed.), *Language, Counter-Memory, Practice*. Ithaca, NY: Cornell University Press, pp. 139–164.

Foucault, M. (1978). *The History of Sexuality*.Vol. 1: *An Introduction*. London: Penguin Books.

Foucault, M. (1980). Truth and power. In C. Gordon (ed.), *Michel Foucault: Power/Knowledge*. New York: Harvester Wheatsheaf, pp. 109–133.

Foucault, M. (1982). Afterword: the subject and power. In H. L. Dreyfus and P. Rabinow, *Michel Foucault: Beyond Structuralism and Hermeneutics*. London: Harvester Press, pp. 208–226.

Foucault, M. (1997). What is critique? In S. Lotringer (ed.), *The Politics of Truth*. Los Angeles: Semiotext(e), pp. 41–81.

Foucault, M. (2000). The birth of social medicine. In J. D. Faubion (ed.), *Michel Foucault: Power*. New York: The New Press, pp. 134–156.

Foucault, M. (2007). *Security, Territory, Population: Lectures at the Collège de France, 1977–1978*. Basingstoke: Palgrave Macmillan.

Foucault, M. (2008). *The Birth of Biopolitics: Lectures at the Collège de France 1978–1979*. Ed. M. Senellart. Basingstoke: Palgrave Macmillan.

Frandsen, M., and Triantafillou, P. (2011). Biopower at the molar level: liberal government and the invigoration of Danish society. *Social Theory and Health*, 9(3): 203–223.

Frohlich, K., Corin, E., and Potvin, L. (2001). A theoretical proposal for the relationship between context and disease. *Sociology of Health and Illness*, 23(6): 776–797.

Gard, M., and Wright, J. (2005). *The Obesity Epidemic*. London: Routledge.

Gately, P. J., Cooke, C. B., Butterly, R. J., Mackreth, P., and Carroll, S. (2000). The effects of a children's summer camp programme on weight loss, with a 10-month follow-up. *International Journal of Obesity Related Metabolic Disorder*, 24: 1445–1452.

Geert-Jørgensen, E. (1963). *Sindssund – sindslidende. Et psykiatrisk strejftog*, Copenhagen: Thaning and Appel.

Geill, C. (1895). *Nogle bemærkninger angående den moderne sindssygebehandling*. Copenhagen: Jacob Lunds Forlag.

Gidley, B. (2007). Sure Start: an upstream approach to reduce health inequalities. In A. Scriven and S. Garman (eds), *Public Health: Social Context and Action*. London: Open University Press, pp. 144–153.

Gloy, V. L., Briel, M., Bhatt, D. L., Kashyap, S. R., Schauer, P. R., Mingrone, G. ... Nordmann, A. J. (2013). Bariatric surgery versus non-surgical treatment for obesity: a systematic review and meta-analysis of randomised controlled trials. *British Medical Journal*, 347: f5934.

Goffman, E. (1961). *Asylums. Essays on the Social Situation of Mental Patients and Other Inmates*. London: Penguin Books.

Gordon, D. (1999). *Inequalities in Health: The Evidence Presented to the Independent Inquiry into Inequalities in Health*. Bristol: Policy Press.

Greco, M. (2008). On the art of life: a vitalist reading of medical humanities. *Sociological Review*, 56(2): 23–45.

Grob, G. N. (1991). *From Asylum to Community: Mental Health Policy in America*. Princeton, NJ: Princeton University Press.

Guardian. (2015). Escalating child health crisis feared due to lack of school nurses. 24 August.

Gudmand-Høyer, M. (2015). Patientpersonen og imødegåelsen af maniodepressive selvmord – en human vending i psykiatrisk praksis. In M. Gudmand-Høyer, S. Raffnsøe, and M. Raffnsøe-Møller (eds), *Den humane vending. En antologi*. Aarhus: Aarhus Universitetsforlag, pp. 161–220.

Ham, C. (2009). *Health Policy in Britain*. 6th edn. Basingstoke: Palgrave Macmillan.

Hansen, E. B. (2012). *Du bestemmer – vægten indeni*. Copenhagen: AKF.

Hansen, T. (2008). Selvudviklingens opkomst i psykiatrien. In S. Brinkmann and P. Triantafillou (eds), *Psykens historier i Danmark. Om forståelsen og styringen af sjælelivet*. Copenhagen: Samfundslitteratur, pp. 71–96.

Harding, C. M., Brooks, G. W., Ashikaka, T., Strauss, J. S., and Breier, A. (1987). The Vermont longitudinal study of persons with severe mental illness, II: long-term outcome of subjects who retrospectively met DSM-III criteria for schizophrenia. *American Journal of Psychiatry*, 144: 727–735.

Harrison, G., Hopper, K., Craig, T., Laska, E., Siegel, C., Wanderling, J., Dube, K. C., Ganev, K., Giel, R., an der Heiden, W., Holmberg, S. K., Janca, A., Lee, P. W., León, C. A., Malhotra, S., Marsella, A. J., Nakane, Y., Sartorius, N., Shen, Y., Skoda, C., Thara, R., Tsirkin, S. J., Varma, V. K., Walsh, D., Wiersma, D. (2001). Recovery from psychotic illness: a 15- and 25-year international follow-up study. *British Journal of Psychiatry*, 178(6): 506–517.

Harting, J., and Assema, P. van. (2011). Exploring the conceptualization of program theories in Dutch community programs: a multiple case study. *Health Promotion International*, 26(1): 23–36.

Henningsen, K., and Dyhrberg, C. N. (2009). Etablering af ny enhed for overvægtige børn og unge. *Diætisten*, 97: 15–17.

Hills, D., Elliott, E., Kowarzik, U., Sullivan, F., Stern, E., Platt, S., and McDaid, D. (2007). *The Big Lottery Fund Healthy Living Centres Programme Final Report*. London: Bridge Consortium, Big Lottery Fund.

HM Government. (2016). *Childhood Obesity: A Plan for Action*. London: The Stationery Office.

Hogg, C. (2009). *Citizens, Consumers and the NHS: Capturing Voices*. Basingstoke: Palgrave Macmillan.

Holloway, F. (2005). *Faculty Report: The Forgotten Need for Rehabilitation in Contemporary Mental Health Services*. London: Faculty of Rehabilitation and Social Psychiatry, Royal College of Psychiatrists.

Holm, J. C. (2015). *Paradigmeskiftet i børneovervægt*. Poster shown at KL Social- og Sundhedspolitisk Forum, 28 May, Aalborg. www.kl.dk/ImageVaultFiles/id_73482/cf_202/Plenum_torsdag_-_plancher_fra_Jens-Christian_Holm.PDF.

Holm, J. C. (2016). Jens-Christian Holm. Forskning. www.jenschristianholm.dk/forskning.

House of Commons Health Committee. (2016). *Public Health post–2013. Second Report of Session 2016–17*. HC 140. London: House of Commons.

Hoyningen-Huene, P., and Wuketits, F. M. (eds) (1989). *Reductionism and Systems Theory in the Life Sciences: Some Problems and Perspectives*. Dordrecht: Springer.

Hugman, R. (1994). Consuming health and welfare. In R. Keat, N. Whiteley and N. Abercrombie (eds), *The Authority of the Consumer*. London: Routledge, pp. 207–222.

Hunt, J. (2017). *Mental health and NHS performance*. Oral statement to Parliament, 9 January. www.gov.uk/government/speeches/mental-health-and-nhs-performance.

Hunter, D. J., Marks, L., and Smith, K. E. (2010). *The Public Health System in England*. Bristol: Policy Press.

Høje-Taastrup Kommune. (2005). *Livsstilsbesøg til 3½-årige og deres familier i Høje-Taastrup Kommune*. Høje-Taastrup: Høje-Taastrup Kommune, Familie- og socialcenteret, Sundhedsplejen.

Idrætspolitisk Forum Fyn. (2010). *Rapport fra møde i Idrætspolitisk Forum Fyn*. 18 March. Odense: Idrætspolitisk Forum Fyn.

Illich, I. (1976). *Medical Nemesis: The Expropriation of Health*. New York: Pantheon Books.

Implement Consulting Group. (2014). *Den Gode Psykiatriske Afdeling – Slutevaluering*. Copenhagen: Sundhedsstyrelsen.

Indenrigs- og Sundhedsministeriet. (2004). *Aftale om strukturreform*. Copenhagen: Indenrigs- og Sundhedsministeriet.

Indenrigs- og Sundhedsministeriet. (2005). *En forstærket indsats mod svær overvægt*. Copenhagen: Indenrigs- og Sundhedsministeriet.

Jackson, N., Waters, E., and Guidelines for Systematic Reviews in Health Promotion and Public Health Taskforce. (2005). Criteria for the systematic review of health promotion and public health interventions. *Health Promotion International*, 20(4): 367–374. http://doi.org/10.1093/heapro/dai022.

Jacobsen, L. (1930). Underlødig-underlødighed. Correspondence. *Ugeskrift for læger*, 50(11 December): 1183–1184.

Jansbøl, K., and Rahbek, A. E. (2013). *Sund Mand – litteraturstudiet*. Copenhagen: KORA.

Jebb, S. A., Aveyard, P. N., and Hawkes, C. (2013). The evolution of policy and actions to tackle obesity in England. *Obesity Reviews*, 14(Suppl. 2): 42–59.

Jensen, P. (2002). *Recovery*. Copenhagen: Videnscenter for Socialpsykiatri.

Johnson, S. (2013). Crisis resolution and home treatment teams: an evolving model. *Articles in Psychiatric Treatment,* 19: 115–123.
Joint Commissioning Panel for Mental Health. (2012). *Guidance for Commissioners of Rehabilitation Services for People with Complex Mental Health Needs 2: Practical Mental Health Commissioning.* London: Joint Commissioning Panel for Mental Health.
Jonasen, V. (2003). *Dansk socialpolitik 1708–2002.* Aarhus: Den Sociale Højskole i Aarhus.
Jones, G. (1986). *Social Hygiene in Twentieth-Century Britain.* London: Croom Helm.
Jones, R., Pyket, J., and Whitehead, M. (2013). *Changing Behaviours: On the Rise of the Psychological State.* Cheltenham: Edward Elgar.
Jørgensen, P. (1998). Ikke at more men at opdrage. In I. Berg-Sørensen and P. Jørgensen (eds), *Een time dagligen. Skoleidræt gennem 200 år.* Odense: Odense Universitetsforlag, pp. 85–150.
Jutel, A. (2005). Weighing health: the moral burden of obesity. *Social Semiotics,* 15(2): 113–125.
Kalidindi, S., Killaspy, H., and Edwards, T. (2012). *Faculty Report: Community Psychosis Services: The Role of Community Mental Health Rehabilitation Teams,* London: Faculty of Rehabilitation and Social Psychiatry, Royal College of Psychiatry.
Kawachi, I., and Kennedy, B. (2002). *The Health of Nations: Why Inequality Is Harmful to Your Health.* New York: New Press.
Kelly, A., and Gamble C. (2005). Exploring the concept of recovery in schizophrenia. *Journal of Psychiatric and Mental Health Nursing,* 12(2): 245–251.
Kelly, M. P., and Charlton, B. (1995). The modern and the postmodern in health promotion. In R. Bunton, S. Nettleton, and R. Burrows (eds), *The Sociology of Health Promotion. Critical Analyses of Consumption, Lifestyle and Risk.* London: Routledge, pp. 78–90.
Kemp, T. (1937). De asociale og forsorgen for dem. *Ugeskrift for Læger,* 99(38): 1009–1014.
King, D. (1999). *In the Name of Liberalism: Illiberal Social Policy in the United States and Britain.* Oxford: Oxford University Press.
Koch, L. (1996). *Racehygiejne i Danmark 1920–56.* Copenhagen: Gyldendal.
Koch, L. (2000). *Tvangssterilisation i Danmark 1929–67.* Copenhagen: Nordisk Forlag.
Kommunernes Landsforening. (2012). *Det nære sundhedsvæsen.* Copenhagen: Kommunernes Landsforening.
Kommunernes Landsforening. (2014a). *Midlet til at nå sundhedsplanens mål er forebyggelsespakkerne.* Copenhagen: Kommunernes Landsforening. www.kl.dk/Aktuelle-temaer/Center-for-Forebyggelse-i-Praksis/Raadgivning/forebyggelsespakkerne_er_midlet/.
Kommunernes Landsforening. (2014b). *Familieorienteret indsats skaber resultater for børn og unge.* Copenhagen: Kommunernes Landsforening. www.kl.dk/Det-nare-sundhedsvasen/Familieorienteret-indsats-skaber-resultater-for-overvagtige-born-og-unge1-id156288/.

Kommunernes Landsforening. (2014c). *Langelands borgere nudges til sundere vaner.* Copenhagen: Kommunernes Landsforening. www.kl.dk/Kommunikation/Langelands-borgere-nudges-til-sundere-vaner-id163221/.

Kommunernes Landsforening. (2015a). *Statusnotat Motion og Bevægelse, Maj 2015.* Copenhagen: Kommunernes Landsforening. www.kl.dk/PageFiles/1300675/Statusnotat%20Motion%20og%20bev%c3%a6gelse.pdf.

Kommunernes Landsforening. (2015b). *Udfordringer og anbefalinger. KL-udspil om sundhed.* Copenhagen: Kommunernes Landsforening. www.kl.dk/ImageVaultFiles/id_75048/cf_202/KL-udspil-_Sammen_om_sundhed_-2015-.PDF.

Kompetencecenter for Rehabilitering og Recovery. (2016). Region Hovedstadens Psykiatri. www.psykiatri-regionh.dk/centre-og-social-tilbud/kompetencecentre/Rehabilitering-og-recovery/Sider/default.aspx (accessed 10 March 2017).

Korsbek, L., Dalum, H. S., Lindschou, J., and Eplov, L. F. (2014). *Illness Management and Recovery Programme for People with Severe Mental Illness (Protocol): The Cochrane Collaboration.* Hoboken, NJ: John Wiley and Sons.

Kragh, J. V. (2008). *Psykiatriens historie i Danmark.* Copenhagen: Hans Reitzels Forlag.

Kromayer, J. (2003). Ny tilgang til psykiatriske diagnoser. *Sygeplejersken*, 27: 12–14.

Kudahl, S. (2012). *Fokus på overvægt begynder at give resultater.* Copenhagen: Kommunernes Landsforening. www.kl.dk/Momentum/Fokus-pa-overvagt-begynder-at-give-resultater-id95463/.

Ladefoged, U. (2014). *Håbet er lysegrønt. Et casestudie i hvordan recoveryorienteret rehabilitering skaber borgerens muligheder for at komme sig på et socialpsykiatrisk botilbud.* Århus: DPU, Århus Universitet.

Laing, R. D. (1960). *The Divided Self: An Existential Study in Sanity and Madness.* Harmondsworth: Penguin Books.

Landsforeningen Af nuværende og tidligere Psykiatribrugere. (2005). *Mennesker med alvorlige psykiske problemer kan komme sig. Hvordan kan det gå til?* Odense: LAP.

Landsforeningen Af nuværende og tidligere Psykiatribrugere. (2010). *Mere end almindelig hensyntagen? Eksempler på inklusion af borgere med psykiske lidelser på arbejdsmarkedet.* Odense: LAP.

Larsen, K. (2014). *Smitstof. Kampen mod sygdom i 1800-tallets Danmark.* Copenhagen: Munksgaard.

Latour, B. (1988). *The Pasteurization of France.* Cambridge, MA: Harvard University Press.

Leichter, H. (1991). *Free to be Foolish: Politics and Health Promotion in the United States and Great Britain.* Princeton, NJ: Princeton University Press.

Leon, D., and Walt, G. (2000). *Poverty, Inequality and Health: An International Perspective.* Oxford: Oxford University Press.

Lindbladh, E., Lyttkens, C. H., Hanson, B. S., and Östergren, P. O. (1998). Equity is out of fashion? An essay on autonomy and health policy in the individualized society. *Social Science and Medicine*, 46(8): 1017–1025.

Local Government Association. (2011). *Communities for Health: Final Evaluation*. London: Local Government Association.
Local Government Association. (2013). *Tackling Obesity: Local Government's New Public Health Role*. London: Local Government Association.
Local Government Association. (2015). *Investing in Our Nation's Future: The First 100 Days of the Next Government. Tackling the Causes and Effects of Obesity.* London: Local Government Association.
Local Government Association and Public Health England. (2014). *Public Health Transformation Nine Months On: Bedding In and Reaching Out*. London: Local Government Association.
Lundbye, O. (1953). Hvorfor mentalhygiejne? *Mentalhygiejne*, 2.
Lupton, D. (1995). *The Imperative of Health: Public Health and the Regulated Body*. London: Sage.
Lupton, D. (2012). *Medicine as Culture: Illness, Disease and the Body*. 3rd edn. London: Sage.
Lützen, K. (1998). *Byen tæmmes. Kernefamilie, sociale reformer og velgørenhed i 1800-tallets København*. Copenhagen: Hans Reitzel.
McCrone, P., Dhanasiri, S., Patel, A., Knapp, M., and Lawton-Smith, S. (2008). *Paying the Price. The Costs of Mental Health Care in England to 2026.* London: King's Fund.
Macintyre, S. (1986). The patterning of health by social position in contemporary Britain: directions for sociological research. *Social Science and Medicine*, 23(4): 393–415.
MacKenzie, D. (1976). Eugenics in Britain. *Social Studies of Science*, 6(3/4): 499–532.
McKeown, T. (1979). *The Role of Medicine: Dream, Mirage, or Nemesis?* 2nd edn. Princeton, NJ: Princeton University Press.
MacLeod, R. M. (1967a). Law, medicine and public opinion: the resistance to compulsory health legislation 1870–1907, part I. *Public Law* (Spring): 107–128.
MacLeod, R. M. (1967b). Law, medicine and public opinion: the resistance to compulsory health legislation 1870–1907, part II. *Public Law* (Autumn): 189–211.
The Marmot Review Team. (2010). *Strategic Review of Health Inequalities in England post-2010. The Marmot Review, Executive Summary*. London: The Marmot Review Team. www.instituteofhealthequity.org/projects/fair-society-healthy-lives-the-marmot-review.
Martin, H. M., and Nielsen, A. (2012). *Livsstilsbehandling af overvægt og fedme*. Copenhagen: DSI.
May, T. (2017). *Prime Minister unveils plans to transform mental health support.* Press Release, 9 January. www.gov.uk/government/news/prime-minister-unveils-plans-to-transform-mental-health-support.
Mayes, C. (2016). *The Biopolitics of Lifestyle: Foucault, Ethics and Healthy Choices*. London: Routledge.
Mental Health Taskforce. (2016). *The Five Year Forward View for Mental Health*. London: Mental Health Taskforce. www.england.nhs.uk/wp-content/uploads/2016/02/Mental-Health-Taskforce-FYFV-final.pdf.

Mik-Meyer, N. (2008). Managing fat bodies: identity regulation between public and private domains. *Critical Social Studies*, 10: 20–35.

Mik-Meyer, N. (2010). Putting the right face on a wrong body: an initial interpretation of fat identities in social work organizations. *Qualitative Social Work*, 9(3): 385–405.

Mik-Meyer, N. (2014). Health promotion viewed in a critical perspective. *Scandinavian Journal of Public Health*, 42(15): 31–35.

Miller, L., Clinton-Davis, S., and Meegan, T. (2014). Journeys to work: the perspective of client and employment specialist of 'Individual Placement and Support' in action. *Mental Health and Social Inclusion*, 18(4): 198–202.

Mills, C. (2013). Biopolitical life. In J. Nilsson and S.-O. Wallenstein (eds), *Foucault, Biopolitics and Governmentality*. Stockholm: Södertörn Philosophical Studies, pp. 73–90.

Ministry of Health. (1929). *Annual Report for the Year 1929*. London: HMSO.

Minkler, M. (1999). Personal responsibility for health? A review of the arguments and the evidence at century's end. *Health Education and Behaviour*, 26(1): 121–141.

Minkler, M. (ed.) (2005). *Community Organizing and Community Building for Health*. New Brunswick, NJ: Rutgers University Press.

Mitchell, R., Dorling, D., and Shaw, M. (2000). *Inequalities in Life and Death: What if Britain Were More Equal?* Bristol: Policy Press.

Møllerhøj, J. (2008). 'Thi sindssygdomme helbredes ikke ved piller og dråber alene' – det psykiatriske sygdomsbegreb og den moralske behandling i dansk psykiatri. In S. Brinkmann and P. Triantafillou (eds), *Psykens historier i Danmark. Om forståelsen og styringen af sjælelivet*. Copenhagen: Samfundslitteratur, pp. 49–70.

Mooney, G. (2012). *The Health of Nations: Towards a New Political Economy*. London: Zed Books.

Moran, M. (1999). *Governing the Health Care State. A Comparative Study of the United Kingdom, the United States and Germany*. Manchester: Manchester University Press.

MoreLife. (2016). *MoreLife. History*. www.more-life.co.uk/Default.aspx?PageName=History (accessed 20 February 2017).

Mountain, D., and Holloway, F. (2007). *Faculty Report. Rehabilitation Services in the UK and Ireland: Current Status and Future Need*. London: Faculty for Rehabilitation and Social Psychiatry, Royal College of Psychiatrists.

Müller, J. P. (1904). *Mit system: 15 minutters dagligt arbejde for sundhedens skyld*. Copenhagen: Tillge.

Munck, V. (1935). Socialhygiejnen og idrætsbevægelsen. *Sund Levevis – Populært tidsskrift for ernæring og hygiejne*, 1(12): 1–4.

Murray, S. (2005). (Un/be)coming out? Rethinking fat politics. *Social Semiotics*, 15(2): 153–163.

Myrdal, A., and Myrdal, G. (1935). *Krise i befolkningsspørgsmålet*. Copenhagen: Martins Forlag.

National Audit Office. (2001). *Tackling Obesity in England*. London: National Audit Office.

National Audit Office. (2014). *Helping People through Mental Health Crisis: The Role of Crisis Resolution and Home Treatment Services*. London: National Audit Office. www.nao.org.uk/report/helping-people-through-mental-health-crisis-the-role-of-crisis-resolution-and-home-treatment-services.
National Child Measurement Programme. (2015). *The National Child Measurement Programme: Pre-measurement Leaflet*. www.gov.uk/government/uploads/system/uploads/attachment_data/file/420760/NCMP_pre-measurement_leaflet_April_2015.pdf.
National Collaborating Centre for Mental Health. (2014). *Psychosis and Schizophrenia in Adults: The NICE Guideline on Treatment and Management*. London: National Institute for Health and Care Excellence.
National Institute for Clinical Excellence. (2002). *Schizophrenia: Core Interventions in the Treatment and Management of Schizophrenia in Primary and Secondary Care*. London: NICE.
National Institute for Health and Care Excellence. (2016). *Transition between Inpatient Mental Health Settings and Community or Care Home Settings*. London: NICE. www.nice.org.uk/guidance/ng53/chapter/Recommendations.
Navarro, V. (1976). *Medicine under Capitalism*. New York: Prodist.
Navarro, V. (2002a). *The Political Economy of Social Inequalities: Consequences for Health and Quality of Life*. Amityville, NY: Baywood Publishing.
Navarro, V. (2002b). A critique of social capital. *International Journal of Health Services*, 32: 423–432.
Navarro, V. (ed.) (2007). *Neoliberalism, Globalization, and Inequalities: Consequences for Health and Quality of Life*. Amityville, NY: Baywood Publishing.
Neale, S., Littlejohns, L. B., Hawe, P., and Sutherland, L. (2008). Great expectations and hard times: developing community indicators in a Healthy Communities Initiative in Canada. *Health Promotion International*, 23(2): 119–126.
NHS Confederation and AllTogetherBetter. (2012). *Community Health Champions: Creating New Relationships with Patients and Communities*. London: NHS Confederation. www.altogetherbetter.org.uk/SharedFiles/Download.aspx?pageid=36andmid=57andfileid=89.
NHS Confederation, Mental Health Network. (2016). *Key facts and trends in mental health. Factsheet, March 2016*. www.nhsconfed.org/~/media/Confederation/Files/Publications/Documents/MHN%20key%20facts%20and%20trends%20factsheet_Fs1356_3_WEB.pdf.
NHS England. (2014a). *Five Year Forward View*. London: NHS. www.england.nhs.uk/wp-content/uploads/2014/10/5yfv-web.pdf.
NHS England. (2014b). Get serious about obesity or bankrupt the NHS. London: NHS. www.england.nhs.uk/2014/09/serious-about-obesity/.
NHS England. (2016). *Thousands benefit as first wave of diabetes prevention programme national rollout is announced*. www.england.nhs.uk/2016/03/nhsdpp/.
NHS Rotherham. (2010). *Weight loss camp. Children celebrate*. www.rotherham.nhs.uk/weight-loss-camp-children-celebrate.htm.
Nielsen, J. (2006a). '... Jeg sad på en stol ude i haven ...'. *Socialpædagogen*, 63(12): 4–6.

Nielsen, J. (2006b). Kunsten af male sig ud af et hjørne. *Socialpædagogen*, 63(4): 17–19.

Nordentoft, M., and Iversen, T. (2010). Rehabilitering ved skizofreni med behandlingsopsøgende teams. In L. F. Eplov, L. Korsbek, L. Petersen and M. Olander (eds), *Psykiatrisk og psykosocial rehabilitering – en recoveryorienteret tilgang*. Copenhagen: Munkgaard Danmark, pp. 131–138.

Odder Kommune. (2016). *Nye tiltag skal hjælpe overvægtige børn*. Oddernettet. www.oddernettet.dk/site.aspx?RoomId=257andNewsId=14744andMenuId=143andlangref=75andSplashId=293.

O'Dowd, A. (2016). Clinicians underwhelmed by 'watered down' childhood obesity strategy. *British Medical Journal*, 354 (22 August).

Olesen, M. S. B. (2015). Peerstøtte sker i øjenhøjde med patienterne. *Sygeplejersken*, 5: 21–24.

Oliver, J. E. (2006). *Fat Politics: The Real Story behind America's Obesity Epidemic*. Oxford: Oxford University Press.

Oliver, T. R. (2006). The politics of public health policy. *Annual Review of Public Health*, 27: 195–233.

Olsen, E. (2016). Retten til selvbestemmelse. www.lap.dk/holdninger/artikler/retten-til-selvbestemmelse/.

Olsen, O. A., and Køppe, S. (1996). *Psykoanalyzen efter Freud*, vol. 1. Copenhagen: Gyldendal.

Olshansky, S. J., Passaro, D. J., Hershow, R. C., Layden, J., and Carnes, B. A. (2005). A potential decline in life expectancy in the United States in the 21st century. *New England Journal of Medicine*, 352(11): 1138–1145.

Osborne, T. (1997). Of health and statecraft. In A. Petersen and R. Bunton (eds), *Foucault, Health and Medicine*. London: Routledge, pp. 173–188.

Osborne, T. (2016). Vitalism as pathos. *Biosemiotics*, 9(2): 185–205.

Parish, R. (1995). Health promotion. Rhetoric and reality. In R. Bunton, S. Nettleton and R. Burrows (eds), *The Sociology of Health Promotion*. London: Routledge, pp. 13–23.

Pearse, I. H., and Crocker, L. H. (2007). *The Peckham Experiment*. London: Routledge.

Pedersen, K. M. (2016). Fedme og sundhedsøkonomi. *Perspektiv* [journal issued by Nordic Sugar], 2. http://perspektiv.nu/da/artikler/fedme-og-sundhedsoekonomi.aspx?PID=71.

Pedersen, L., and Andreassen, L. (2015). *Når dokumentation understøtter recovery. Fem undersøgelsers svar på spørgsmålet: 'Hvad skal der til for at dokumentation giver mening – og understøtter den enkelte persons muligheder for at komme videre i livet'*. Interessegruppen for dokumentation og forskning i Dansk Selskab for Psykosocial Rehabilitering. Copenhagen: Dansk Selskab for Psykosocial Rehabilitering.

Petersen, A. (1996). The 'healthy' city, expertise, and the regulation of space. *Health and Space*, 2(3): 157–165.

Petersen, A., and Bunton, R. (1997). *Foucault: Health and Medicine*. London: Routledge.

Power, P., Smith, J. Shiers, D., and Roberts, G. (2006). Early intervention in first-episode psychosis and its relevance to rehabilitation psychiatry. In G. Roberts, S. Davenport, F. Holloway, and T. Tattan (eds), *Enabling Recovery: The Principles and Practice of Rehabilitation Psychiatry*, Trowbridge: Cromwell Press, pp. 127–146.

Public Health England. (2014). *Everybody Active, Every Day: An Evidence-Based Approach to Physical Activity*. London: Public Health England.
Public Health England. (2015a). *Social Marketing Strategy 2014–2017: One Year On*. London: Public Health England.
Public Health England. (2015b). *National Child Measurement Programme Operational Guidance 2015 to 2016*. London: Public Health England.
Public Health England. (2016). *About Obesity: UK and Ireland Prevalence and Trends*. London Public Health England. www.noo.org.uk/NOO_about_obesity/adult_obesity/UK_prevalence_and_trends.
Public Health England, Department of Health, SAPHNA, Royal College of Nursing, CPHVA, and Unite. (2014). *Health Visiting and School Nursing Programmes: Supporting Implementation of the New Service Model: Health Visiting and School Nursing Partnership – Pathways for Supporting Health Visitor and School Nurse Interface and Improved Partnership Working*. London: Public Health England.
Rådgivende Sociologer. (2014). *Shared care i psykiatrien. En evaluering af projektet*. Copenhagen: Rådgivende Sociologer ApS.
Raffnsøe, S., Gudmand-Høyer, M., and Thaning, M. S. (2016). *Michel Foucault: A Research Companion*. Basingstoke: Palgrave Macmillan.
Rawlinson, K., and Johnston, C. (2016). Decision to deny surgery to obese patients is like 'racial discrimination'. *Guardian*, 3 September.
Rayner, E. (1990). *The Independent Mind in British Psychoanalysis*. London: Free Association Books.
Regeringen. (2002). *Sund hele livet – de nationale mål og strategier for folkesundheden 2002–2010*. Copenhagen: Regeringen.
Regeringen. (2014). *Sundere liv for alle. Nationale mål for danskernes sundhed de næste 10 år*. Copenhagen: Sundhedsministeriet.
Region Hovedstadens Psykiatri. (2014). 'Temanummer: Recovery', *PsykiatriNyt*, May 2014.
Region Hovedstadens Psykiatri. (2015a). *Akuthjælp rykker ud til borgerne*. www.psykiatri-regionh.dk/presse-og-nyt/pressemeddelelser-og-nyheder/Nyheder-og-pressemeddelelser/Sider/Akuthjælp-rykker-hjem-til-borgerne.aspx.
Region Hovedstadens Psykiatri. (2015b). *Brugerfortællinger*. www.psykiatri-regionh.dk/undersoegelse-og-behandling/Recovery/Brugerfortaellinger/Sider/default.aspx?rhKeywords=brugerfort%C3%A6llinger.
Region Hovedstadens Psykiatri. (2015c). *Fakta: Hvad er recovery?* www.psykiatri-regionh.dk/undersoegelse-og-behandling/Recovery/Om-recovery/Sider/Fakta-hvad-er-recovery.aspx.
Region Hovedstadens Psykiatri. (2015d). *Om recovery*. www.psykiatri-regionh.dk/undersoegelse-og-behandling/Recovery/Om-recovery/Sider/default.aspx.
Region Hovedstadens Psykiatri. (2015e). *Personlige drømme og mål*. www.psykiatri-regionh.dk/Kvalitet-og-udvikling/skolen-for-recovery/kurser/Sider/Personlige-dr%C3%B8mme-og-m%C3%A5l.aspx.
Region Hovedstadens Psykiatri. (2015f). *Personlige mål i behandlingsplanen*. www.psykiatri-regionh.dk/undersoegelse-og-behandling/Recovery/Recoveryprojekter-og-tiltag-i-RHP/Sider/Personlige-maal-i-behandlingsplanen.aspx.

Region Hovedstadens Psykiatri. (2015g). *Recovery – et liv i forandring.* www.psykiatri-regionh.dk/Kvalitet-og-udvikling/skolen-for-recovery/kurser/Sider/Recovery---et-liv-i-forandring.aspx.

Region Hovedstadens Psykiatri. (2015h). *Recoverymentorer.* www.psykiatri-regionh.dk/centre-og-social-tilbud/kompetencecentre/Rehabilitering-og-recovery/Recovery-mentorer_i_Region_Hovedstadens_Psykiatri/Sider/default.aspx.

Region Hovedstadens Psykiatri. (2015i). *Recoveryværktøjer og tiltag.* www.psykiatri-regionh.dk/undersoegelse-og-behandling/Recovery/Recoveryprojekter-og-tiltag-i-RHP/Sider/default.aspx.

Region Hovedstadens Psykiatri. (2015j). *Styrk dit netværk og dine relationer.* www.psykiatri-regionh.dk/Kvalitet-og-udvikling/skolen-for-recovery/kurser/Sider/Styrk-dit-netv%C3%A6rk-og-dine-relationer.aspx.

Region Hovedstadens Psykiatri. (2015k). *Tag kontrollen i dit liv.* www.psykiatri-regionh.dk/Kvalitet-og-udvikling/skolen-for-recovery/nyheder-fra-skolen-for-Recovery/Sider/P%C3%A5-kursus-i-recovery.aspx.

Region Hovedstadens Psykiatri. (2016). *Recovery: håb og muligheder for at komme sig.* www.psykiatri-regionh.dk/undersoegelse-og-behandling/Recovery/Sider/default.aspx.

Region Sjælland. (2014). *Gennembrud i kommuners behandling af børn med overvægt.* www.regionsjaelland.dk/nyheder/Sider/Gennembrud-i-kommuners-behandling-af-boern-med-overvaegt.aspx.

Reiter, P. J. (1950). *Vejledning i psykotherapeutisk teknik.* Copenhagen: Westermann.

Rigsrevisionen. (2013). *Beretning til Statsrevisorerne om borgerrettet forebyggelse på sundhedsområdet.* Copenhagen: Rigsrevisionen.

Roberts, G., and Wolfson, P. (2006). New directions in rehabilitation: learning from the recovery movement. In G. Roberts, S. Davenport, F. Holloway and T. Tattan (eds), *Enabling Recovery: The Principles and Practice of Rehabilitation Psychiatry.* Trowbridge: Cromwell Press, pp. 18–38.

Roberts, G., Davenport, S., Holloway, F., and Tattan, T. (eds) (2006a). *Enabling Recovery: The Principles and Practice of Rehabilitation Psychiatry.* Trowbridge: Cromwell Press.

Roberts, G., Davenport, S., Holloway, F., and Tattan. T. (2006b). Preface. In G. Roberts, S. Davenport, F. Holloway, and T. Tattan (eds), *Enabling Recovery: The Principles and Practice of Rehabilitation Psychiatry.* Trowbridge: Cromwell Press, pp. xv–3.

Rockhill, B. (2001). The privatization of risk. *American Journal of Public Health,* 91: 365–368.

Rønholt, H., and Peitersen, B. (2005). *Idrætsundervisning – en grundbog i idrætsdidaktik.* Copenhagen: Forlaget Hovedland.

Rose, G. (2001). Sick individuals and sick populations. *International Journal of Epidemiology,* 30(3): 427–432.

Rose, N. (1989). *Governing the Soul: The Shaping of the Private Self.* London: Routledge.

Rose, N. (1999). *Powers of Freedom: Reframing Political Thought.* Cambridge: Cambridge University Press.

Rose, N. (2006). *The Politics of Life Itself: Biomedicine, Power and Subjectivity in the Twenty-First Century*. Princeton, NJ: Princeton University Press.

Ross, T. (2012). David Cameron ordered to stop saying NHS spending is up. *Daily Telegraph*, 4 December.

Royal College of Paediatrics and Child Health. (2015). *Tackling England's Childhood Obesity Crisis. A Report by the Royal College of Paediatrics and Child Health to Inform the Development of the UK Government's Childhood Obesity Strategy*. London: Royal College of Paediatrics and Child Health.

Rubow, P. (1930). Minderwertigkeit. *Ugeskrift for Læger*, 48: 1109–1010.

Salter, B. (2007). Governing UK medical performance: a struggle for policy dominance. *Health Policy*, 82: 263–275.

Schwartz, J. (1999). *Cassandra's Daughter: A History of Psychoanalysis*. London: Penguin Books.

Secretary of State for Health. (1992). *The Health of the Nation: A Strategy for Health in England*. London: HMSO.

Secretary of State for Health. (1999a). *Saving Lives: Our Healthier Nation*. London: The Stationery Office.

Secretary of State for Health. (1999b). *A National Service Framework for Mental Health: Modern Standard and Services Models*. London: Department of Health.

Secretary of State for Health. (2010). *Healthy Lives, Healthy People: Our Strategy for Public Health in England*. London: Department of Health.

Secretary of State for Health. (2011). *Healthy Lives, Healthy People: Update and Way Forward*. Cm 8134. London: HMSO.

Selmer, H. (1846). *Almindelige grundsætninger for dårevæsenets indretning som fast resultat af videnskab og erfaring fremstillet for det større publicum af H. Selmer*. Copenhagen: BUH.

Sholl, J., and De Block, A. (2015). Towards a critique of normalization: Boore and Canguilhem. In *Medicine and Society. New Perspectives in Continental Philosophy*. Dordrecht: Springer, pp. 141–158.

Short, A., Phillips, R., Nugus, P., Dugdale, P., and Greenfield, D. (2015). Developing an inter-organizational community-based health network: an Australian investigation. *Health Promotion International*, 30(4): 868–880.

Shorter, E. (1997). *A History of Psychiatry: From the Era of the Asylum to the Age of Prozac*. New York: John Wiley.

SIND. (2015). *SINDs Landsmøde 2015*. www.sind.dk/6storage/113/0/sinds_handleplaner_2015_til_2018.pdf.

SIND. (2016). *SIND ambassadører*. www.sind.dk/ambassadoerer.

Slade, M. (2013). *100 Ways to Support Recovery: A Guide for Mental Health Professionals*. London: Rethink Mental Illness/Rethink.org.

Socialforskningsinstitutet. (2004). *Det kommunale råderum – Kvalitet effektivitet og forskellighed i velfærdsydelserne*. Denmark: Social Forskning.

Socialministeriet and Indenrigs- og Sundhedsministeriet. (2005). *Fælles værdier i indsatsen for mennesker med en sindslidelse. Respekt, faglighed, ansvar*. Copenhagen: Socialministeriet and Indenrigs- og Sundhedsministeriet.

Socialstyrelsen. (2013). *Mennesker med psykiske vanskeligheder. Sociale indsatser der virker*. Odense: Socialstyrelsen.

Sønderborg Nyt. (2015). Ny overvægtsklinik skal hjælpe tykke og fede børn. www.sønderborgnyt.dk/ny-overvaegtsklinik-skal-hjaelpe-tykke-og-fede-boern/.

South, J., White, J., and Gamsu, M. (2013). *People-Centred Public Health*. Bristol: Policy Press.

Starr, P. (1982). *The Social Transformation of American Medicine*. New York: Basic Books.

Statens Institut for Folkesundhed. (2013). *Danskernes sundhed. Tal fra den nationale sundhedsprofil*. Odense: Statens Institut for Folkesundhed. www.sundhedsprofil2010.dk/overvaegt-og-undervaegt/.

Statens Institut for Folkesundhed. (2016). *Databasen Børns Sundhed*. Odense: Statens Institut for Folkesundhed. www.si-folkesundhed.dk/Links/Databasen%20B%C3%B8rns%20Sundhed/Om%20databasen.aspx.

Statsministeriet. (2001). *Statsminister Poul Nyrup Rasmussens tale den 26. marts 2001 ved jubilæumskonference om Psykiatriens 25 år i amterne*. www.stm.dk/_p_7732.html.

Storm, L. K., Madsen, S., and Ibsen, B. (2012). *Evaluering af projekt Grib Chancen Projekt om fysisk aktivitet for børn og unge i et partnerskab mellem kommuner og foreninger på Fyn*. Odense: Institut for Idræt og Biomekanik, Syddansk Universitet.

Strøm, C. (2012). Succes med ny tilgang til svær overvægt. *Ugeskrift for Læger*, 174(18): 1198–1199.

Sund By Netværket. (2016). Sund By Netværket. Medlemmer. http://sund-by-net.dk/medlemmer.

Sundhedsministeriet. (1989a). *Regeringens forebyggelsesprogram. Dokumentationsdel*. Copenhagen: Sundhedsministeriet.

Sundhedsministeriet. (1989b). *Regeringens forebyggelsesprogram. Programdel*. Copenhagen: Sundhedsministeriet.

Sundhedsministeriet. (1999). *Regeringens folkesundhedsprogram 1999–2008*. Copenhagen: Sundhedsministeriet.

Sundhedsministeriet and Socialministeriet. (2001). *Rapport fra udvalget vedrørende bedre samspil mellem tilbuddene i psykiatrien og socialpsykiatrien*. Copenhagen: Sundhedsministeriet and Socialministeriet.

Sundhedsstyrelsen. (1999). *Konsekvenser af overvægt og fedme*. Copenhagen: Sundhedsstyrelsen.

Sundhedsstyrelsen. (2003). *Oplæg til national handlingsplan mod svær overvægt – Forslag til løsninger og perspektiver*. Copenhagen: Sundhedsstyrelsen, Center for Forebyggelse.

Sundhedsstyrelsen. (2005). *Terminologi. Forebyggelse, sundhedsfremme og folkesundhed*. Copenhagen: Sundhedsstyrelsen.

Sundhedsstyrelsen. (2009). *National strategi for psykiatri*. August 2009. Copenhagen: Sundhedsstyrelsen.

Sundhedsstyrelsen. (2012a). *Forebyggelsespakke – Fysisk aktivitet*. Copenhagen: Sundhedsstyrelsen.

Sundhedsstyrelsen. (2012b). *Forebyggelsespakke – Hygiejne*. Copenhagen: Sundhedsstyrelsen.

Sundhedsstyrelsen. (2012c). *Forebyggelsespakke – Tobak*. Copenhagen: Sundhedsstyrelsen.

Sundhedsstyrelsen. (2012d). *Forebyggelsespakke – Alkohol*. Copenhagen: Sundhedsstyrelsen.
Sundhedsstyrelsen. (2012e). *Sammenfattende evaluering af projekterne i satspuljen: Kommunernes plan mod overvægt blandt børn og unge*. Copenhagen: Sundhedsstyrelsen.
Sundhedsstyrelsen. (2013). *Forebyggelsespakke – Overvægt*. Copenhagen: Sundhedsstyrelsen.
Sundhedsstyrelsen. (2014a). *Satspuljeopslag: Forsøg med ambulante akutteams i den regionale psykiatri*. Copenhagen: Sundhedsstyrelsen. http://sundhedsstyrelsen.dk/da/soeg?q=nice.
Sundhedsstyrelsen. (2014b). *Puljer: Erfaringer med peer støtte*. Copenhagen: Sundhedsstyrelsen.
Sundhedsstyrelsen. (2014c). *Danskernes Sundhed – Den Nationale Sundhedsprofil 2013*. Copenhagen: Sundhedsstyrelsen. http://sundhedsstyrelsen.dk/~/media/1529A4BCF9C64905BAC650B6C45B72A5.ashx.
Svendsen, O. L., Heitmann, B. L., Mikkelsen, K. L., Raben, A., Ryttig, K. R., Sørensen, T. I. A. ... Toubro, S. (2001). *Fedme i Danmark. En rapport fra Dansk Task Force on Obesity*. Klaringsrapport 8. Copenhagen: Dansk Selskab for Adipositasforskning.
Syddjurs Kommune. (2015). *Behandling af svært overvægtige børn og unge. 'Holbæk Modellen'.* www.syddjurs.dk/sites/default/files/PDF/Holb%C3%A6k-modellen.pdf.
Sygehuse and Beredskab. (2014). *Udvikling af modelafdelinger: Den Gode Psykiatriske Afdeling*. Copenhagen: Sygehuse and Beredskab.
Taylor, M. (2007). Community participation in the real world: opportunities and pitfalls in new governance spaces. *Urban Studies*, 44 (2): 297–317.
Teglgaard, K. (2004). *Sundhed – en del af DGIs formålsparagraf*. Argument proposed by member of DGI executive board, Karen Teglgaard. Unpublished memo.
Thaler, R. H., and Sunstein, C. (2008). *Nudge: Improving Decisions about Health, Wealth and Happiness*. New Haven, CT: Yale University Press.
Thomson, M. (1998). *The Problem of Mental Deficiency: Eugenics, Democracy, and Social Policy in Britain c. 1870–1959*. Oxford: Oxford University Press.
Tidsskriftet Outsideren. (2016). De personlige erfaringer bliver ekspertviden. 7 April, p. 384.
Tønder, E. S.. (2014). Kronik: patienterfaringer som ny ressource i psykiatrien. *Kristeligt Dagblad*. 6 February.
Topor, A. (2003). *Recovery. At komme sig efter alvorlige psykiske lidelser*. Copenhagen: Hans Reitzels Forlag.
Topor, A. (2005). *Mennesker med alvorlige psykiske lidelser kan komme sig. Hvordan kan det gå til?* Odense: Landsforeningen af nuværende Og tidligere Psykiatribrugere.
Townsend, P., Davidson, N., and Whitehead, M. (1988). *The Black Report and the Health Divide*. Harmondsworth: Penguin Books.
Triantafillou, P. (2012). *New Forms of Governing: A Foucauldian Inspired Analysis*. Basingstoke: Palgrave Macmillan.

Triantafillou, P. (2017). *Neoliberal Power and Public Management Reforms*. Manchester: Manchester University Press.

Trostle, J. A. (1988). Medical compliance as ideology. *Social Science and Medicine*, 27(12): 1299–1308.

Tuke, S. (1813). *Description of the Retreat. An Institution near York for Insane Persons of the Society of Friends Containing an Account of Its Origin and Progress, the Modes of Treatment, and a Statement of Cases*. York: W. Alexander.

Turner, B. (2008). *The Body and Society: Explorations in Social Theory*. 3rd edn. London: Sage.

Ulijaszek, S. J., and McLennan, A. K. (2016). Framing obesity in UK policy from the Blair years, 1997–2015: the persistence of individualistic approaches despite overwhelming evidence of societal and economic factors, and the need for collective responsibility. *Obesity Reviews*, 17: 397–411.

Valiér, C. (1998). Psychoanalysis and crime in Britain during the interwar years. In Jon Vagg and Tim Newburn (eds), *The British Criminology Conferences: Selected Proceedings*. Vol. 1: *Emerging Themes in Criminology*. Papers from the British Criminology Conference, Loughborough University, 18–21 July 1995.

Vallgårda, S. (1989). Hospitals and the poor in Denmark, 1750–1880. *Scandinavian Journal of History*, 13: 95–105.

Vallgårda, S. (2003). *Folkesundhed som politik – Danmark og Sverige fra 1930 til i dag*. Aarhus: Aarhus Universitetsforlag.

van Baal, P. H. M., Polder, J. J., de Wit, G. A., Hoogenveen, R. T., Feenstra, T. L., Boshuizen, H. C., and Brouwer, W. F. (2008). Lifetime medical costs of obesity: prevention no cure for increasing health expenditure. *PLoS Medicine*, 5(2): e29.

Vangaard, T. (1955). Freud i dag. *Politikens Kronik*, 8 August.

Villadsen, K., and Dean, M. (2012). State-phobia, civil society, and a certain vitalism. *Constellations*, 19(3): 401–420.

Villadsen, K., and Wahlberg, A. (2015). The government of life: managing populations, health and scarcity. *Economy and Society*, 44(1): 1–17. doi.org/10.1080/03085147.2014.983831.

Viner, R. M., Roche, E., Maguire, S. A., and Nicholls, D. E. (2010). Childhood protection and obesity: framework for practice. *British Medical Journal*, 341: c3074.

Vucina, N. (2014). *Mind the Body. A Genealogy of Danish Preventive Health and Health Promotion in the Interwar Period and Turn of the Millennium*. PhD dissertation, Department of Society and Globalisation, Roskilde University.

Vucina, N., and Triantafillou, P. (2009). HIV, constructionism and biopower. *Distinktion – Tidsskrift for Samfundsteori*, 18: 29–46.

Wahlberg, A. (2016). Assessing vitality: infertility and 'good life' in urban China. In J. Yorke (ed.), *The Right to Life and the Value of Life*. London: Routledge, pp. 371–396.

Wakefield, S. E. L., and Poland, B. (2005). Family, friend or foe? Critical reflections on the relevance and role of social capital in health promotion and community development. *Social Science and Medicine*, 60(12): 2819–2832.

Walker, C., and Cannon, G. (1985). *The Food Scandal: What's Wrong with the British Diet and How to Put it Right*. London: Century.

Walker, L. L. M., Gately, P. J., Bewick, B. M., and Hill, A. J. (2003). Children's weight-loss camps: psychological benefit or jeopardy? *International Journal of Obesity*, 27: 748–475.
Walt, G., Shiffman, J., Schneider, H., Murray, S. F., Brugha, R., and Gilson, L. (2008). 'Doing' health policy analysis: methodological and conceptual reflections and challenges. *Health, Policy and Planning*, 23(5): 308–317.
Wanless, D. (2004). *Securing Good Health for the Whole Population: Final Report*. London: HM Treasury.
Wilken, J.-P., and den Hollænder, D. (2008). *Rehabilitering og Recovery – En integreret tilgang*. Copenhagen: Akademisk Forlag.
Wilkinson, R. G. (2005). *The Impact of Inequality: How to Make Sick Societies Healthier*. New York: New Press.
Wilson, J. Q. (1980). *The Politics of Regulation*. New York: Basic Books.
Wing, J. K., and Morris, B. (eds) (1981). *Handbook of Psychiatric Rehabilitation Practice*. Oxford: Oxford University Press.
World Health Organization. (1982). *Prevention of Coronary Heart Disease: Report of a WHO Expert Committee*. Technical Report Series 678. Geneva: WHO.
World Health Organization. (1986). *Ottawa Charter for Health Promotion*. Vol. WHO/HPR/HE. Geneva: WHO.
World Health Organization. (1995). *Psychosocial Rehabilitation. A Consensus Statement*. Geneva: Division of Mental Health and Prevention of Substance Abuse, WHO.
World Health Organization. (1998). *Health 21: Health for All in the 21st Century*. Geneva: WHO, European Region.
World Health Organization. (2001). *The World Health Report. Mental Health: New Understanding, New Hope*. Geneva: WHO.
World Health Organization. (2007). *Community mental health services will lessen social exclusion, says WHO*. www.who.int/mediacentre/news/notes/2007/np25/en/.
World Health Organization. (2016). *Obesity and overweight*. www.who.int/mediacentre/factsheets/fs311/en/.
World Health Organization, Regional Office for Europe. (1985). *Targets for Health for All*. Copenhagen: WHO, European Region.
World Health Organization, Regional Office for Europe. (2006). *European Charter on Counteracting Obesity*. Copenhagen: WHO, European Region. www.euro.who.int/__data/assets/pdf_file/0009/87462/E89567.pdf.
Zweiniger-Bargielowska, I. (2005). The culture of the abdomen: obesity and reducing in Britain, circa 1900–1939. *Journal of British Studies*, 44(2): 239–273.
Zweiniger-Bargielowska, I. (2006). Building a British superman: physical culture in interwar Britain. *Journal of Contemporary History*, 1(4): 595–610.

Index

Antonovsky, Aaron 40
archaeology 23
Armstrong, David 18

bariatric surgery 64, 71
Behavioural Insights Team 45
behavioural psychology 44, 70
   see also nudging
Bergson, Henri 9
biobank 94
biopower/biopolitics/biopolitical
   interventions 2, 7–9, 11, 19, 21,
   25, 32–39, 56–57, 61–62,
   90–93, 97, 114, 130, 138,
   141–144
Bleuler, Eugen 106
BMI *see* Body Mass Index
Body Mass Index (BMI) 60, 73, 79, 81,
   83–85, 94, 134, 144
Brüel, Oluf 116–117

Canguilhem, Georges 9
capitalism 16
Change4Life 21, 43, 69
clinical approach 105
CMHT *see* community mental
   health teams
Coalition government (Britain) 43–46,
   53, 55, 59, 66, 68–69, 71–72,
   110, 139
coercion 3, 6, 37, 48, 73, 112, 139
   see also coercive methods
coercive methods 2, 3, 25, 35, 64, 101
   see also coercion

Commission of Preventive Health
   Care 49
Communities for Health
   programme 53
Community Health Councils 50
Community Health Educator
   programmes 52
community mental health teams
   (CMHT) 102, 110, 112–113
community rehabilitation teams 110
Competence Centre for Rehabilitation
   and Recovery 124, 127
Conrad, Peter 18
Conservative government (Britain)
   41–45, 63–64, 66, 69
costs
   economic/fiscal 1, 4–5, 7, 39–40,
      46, 54, 59, 64, 71, 73, 87, 96
   critique 13–14, 17, 19, 22–28, 72, 80,
      82, 96, 116, 129, 137, 140, 143
curative approaches/curative strategies
   2, 7, 35–39, 42, 45–49, 51, 57,
   66, 68, 107, 113, 133, 138, 140

Danish Gymnastics and Sports
   Association (DGI) 55–56
Danish Institute for Clinical
   Epidemiology 47
Dean, Mitchell 9, 22, 25–26, 34, 96
DGI *see* Danish Gymnastics and
   Sports Association
Diagnostic and Statistical Manual
   of Mental Disorders (DSM)
   106–107, 113

Index

dispositive 21
DSM *see* Diagnostic and Statistical Manual of Mental Disorders

economic incentives 44, 69
empowerment
   citizens/patient 52, 114
   community 20, 23, 29, 58, 77, 109, 134
      see also environment: institutional
environment
   institutional 10–11, 21, 57–58, 60, 91, 134, 140–141
      see also community empowerment
   physical 2, 4, 35, 37–38, 47, 49–50, 57, 70, 139
epidemiology
   knowledge 25–26, 34, 140
   studies/surveys 37, 41, 47–48, 57, 64, 80, 83–85, 97, 142
eugenics
   negative 35, 38, 57, 81–82, 139
   positive 62, 80, 82
Evans, Bethan 60, 66, 77, 135–136
expert
   knowledge 7, 11–12, 21, 25, 32, 61, 109, 140
   patient 105
expertise 18–19, 25, 32, 89, 99, 100, 105, 113, 115–116, 126–127, 130, 140, 145
   see also expert knowledge
extra-clinical approach 116, 119–122

facilitator 43, 52, 131
Faculty of Rehabilitation and Social Psychiatry 109
FitFarms 75
Foresight analysis 65–67, 72
Foucault, Michel 2, 6–8, 11, 13, 19–20, 22–27, 32, 77, 116, 131, 135, 142
France 28, 101, 117
Freud, Sigmund 118

genealogy 22–24, 29, 61, 114
genetic screening 94–95
Germany 36
Goffman, Erving 100, 129
governmentality 7–8, 20, 25–26, 32, 130, 142–143
   see also political rationality/ies
governmentalization 58, 140
gymnastics 4, 82, 85
   movement 56, 90, 134

health expenditures 42, 73, 142
Health of the Nation – A Strategy for England, The 63
Healthy Cities Network 46
Healthy Living Centre programme 51, 65
Healthy Weight, Healthy Lives 67
hereditary approaches 38, 63, 94, 106–107
   see also heritage
heritage (biological) 97, 107
   see also hereditary approaches
Holbæk model 93–95
home visits 52, 67
House of Commons Health Committee 68, 72

ICD *see* international classification of mental illness model
Individual and Placement Support programme 111
industrialization 34
information campaign 46, 54, 62–63, 68, 76–77, 134–135
international classification of mental illness model (ICD) 106, 113
interview 31, 118

Joint Commissioning Panel for Mental Health 112

Koch, Lene 38, 81
Kommunernes Landsforening (Local Government Denmark) 88–89, 94, 98

Laing, Ronald D. 102
laissez-faire 28, 44, 121
LAP *see* National Association of Present and Former Psychiatry Users
lifestyle 4–5, 7–8, 10–12, 14, 16–17, 21, 39–57, 63, 66–69, 72, 74–77, 79–80, 84–87, 89–90, 94–95, 107, 111, 134–135, 139–141, 145

Local Government Association 30, 53, 71–72, 74, 135
Lupton, Deborah 20

Marmot Report (Fair Society, Healthy Lives) 44
method 11, 14, 22–23, 28–31, 44, 81, 91, 100–101, 120, 123, 126, 129, 140
MIND 102, 123, 126
moral treatment 100–101, 117–119, 136–137
Müller, Jørgen Peter 82
Myrdal, Alva and Gunnar 38, 81

NACNE *see* National Advisory Committee on Nutrition Education
National Advisory Committee on Nutrition Education (NACNE) 63
National Association of Present and Former Psychiatry Users (LAP) 125–126, 128, 130
National Board of Health (Denmark) 116, 122–123, 126–127, 130
National Institute for Health and Care Excellence (NICE) 103, 111
National Child Measurement Programme 73–74
National Collaborating Centre for Mental Health 106, 108–111, 137
Navarro, Vicente 16, 18
neoliberalism/neoliberal government 8, 20–21, 26–28, 45–46, 77, 96–97, 131–132, 141–143
  constructivist neoliberalism 8, 28, 45–46, 77, 96–97, 141–143
  critical neoliberalism 28, 141
  Ordo-Liberalen 27
New Labour 42–45, 50, 52–53, 59, 64, 66–69, 72, 109–110
NHS England 71, 76, 112
NICE *see* National Institute for Health and Care Excellence
nudging 44–45, 58n.2, 69, 77, 90, 98n.2, 134, 143–144
  see also behavioural psychology

objectification/objectifying knowledge 31, 60, 117, 136, 140
Osborne, Thomas 2, 9, 37

pathos (of life) 9, 144
pedagogic/pedagogical knowledge 24–25, 32, 91, 97, 134, 140
pedagogy 140
  see also pedagogic/pedagogical knowledge
Petersen, Alan 20–21
policy process analysis 14–15, 32
political economy and ideology studies 15–17, 32
political rationality/ies 8, 11–12, 20, 30, 45, 60–61, 64, 96, 99, 115, 139, 141, 143
  see also governmentality
Portman Clinic 101
positive psychology 94
predisposition 70, 97, 107
Prevention Package for Obesity 87–88
problematization 12, 24, 31, 79–80, 114, 131
psychiatry 5–6, 109, 114–115, 121–124, 126, 137
  psychiatric treatment 115–119, 122, 126, 129
  psychiatric diagnoses 120
  psychiatric patients 11–12, 116, 120–121, 125–126
psychoanalysis 101–102, 117–119

rational choice 69, 72
regime of truth 24–25
Region Hovedstadens Psykiatri (Psychiatric Services for the Capital Region) 120, 123–125, 127–128
rehabilitation 11–12, 71, 103, 109–110, 121–122, 124, 127–130, 137
risk 4–5, 10, 13, 19–20, 28, 46, 48–49, 56–57, 60, 63, 67–68, 80–81, 84–85, 88–89, 91, 105, 134, 136, 139, 141, 144
Rose, Nikolas 7, 25–26, 102, 109, 143

Royal College of Psychiatrists 101, 105, 109, 130, 137
Rubow, Paul 116–117

savoir-faire 84–85
schizophrenia 6, 23, 28–29, 102–103, 106–108, 113, 119–120, 122, 124, 129, 137
self-government/self-governing 23, 57, 64, 101, 116, 121, 129, 131, 136, 141–142
  see also self-steering (individual); self-subjectification
self-steering (individual) 7–8, 26–28, 50, 57, 96, 99–100, 113, 118, 126, 131, 137, 143
  see also self-government; self-subjectification
self-subjectification 60, 131, 136
  see also self-government; self-steering (individual)
shared care 122–123, 130
SIND 123, 125–127, 130
Slade, Mike 104–105, 128
social democratic parties 39
Social Democrats 48, 55, 81
Social Marketing Unit, the 70
social welfarism 26, 30, 36, 38, 45, 83, 143
sociological critique of health promotion 17–19, 25
somatic 4, 28
sovereign power/sovereign state power 2–3, 25
structural reform (Denmark, 2007) 47, 54–55, 87, 89–90, 121–122, 130, 132n.1, 135
subjection 80

Topor, Alain 119–120, 126, 128–129, 137
totalizing 21, 46, 96
Triantafillou, Peter 8, 21, 24, 28, 45, 47–48, 58n.1, 96, 141–142
Tuke, William 100–101, 117
Turner, Bryan 20

urbanization 34

Vallgårda, Signild 38, 46
Vermont longitudinal study 107
vitalism/vitalist 9, 25
  optimistic 8–9, 78, 97, 131, 136, 141, 144
voluntary organizations 3–4, 39, 41, 56, 58, 60, 62, 71, 86, 91, 109, 134
Vucina, Naja 5, 24, 31, 56, 81–82, 85, 90, 92

Wahlberg, Ayo 9
WHO see World Health Organization
World Health Organization (WHO) 3–4, 6, 40–41
  Health for All strategy 3, 29, 134, 141
  Ottawa charter 3, 39, 46, 57

EU authorised representative for GPSR:
Easy Access System Europe, Mustamäe tee 50,
10621 Tallinn, Estonia
gpsr.requests@easproject.com